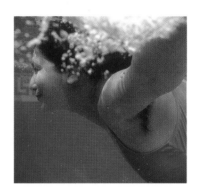

Aqua Yoga
for pregnancy

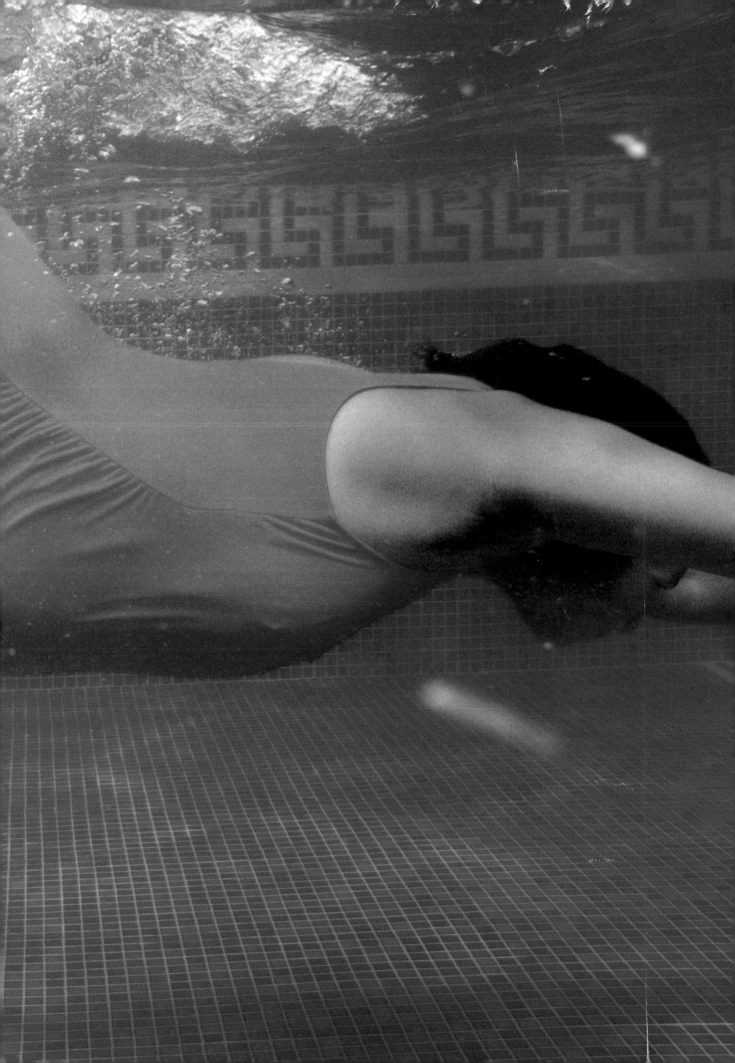

Aqua Yoga for pregnancy

harmonizing exercises in water for health and
fitness in pregnancy, and to get ready for birth

françoise barbira freedman

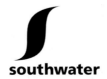

southwater

This edition is published by Southwater

Southwater is an imprint of Anness Publishing Ltd
Hermes House, 88–89 Blackfriars Road, London SE1 8HA
tel. 020 7401 2077; fax 020 7633 9499
www.southwaterbooks.com; info@anness.com

© Anness Publishing Ltd 2000, 2003

UK agent: The Manning Partnership Ltd
6 The Old Dairy, Melcombe Road, Bath BA2 3LR
tel. 01225 478444; fax 01225 478440; sales@manning-partnership.co.uk

UK distributor: Grantham Book Services Ltd
Isaac Newton Way, Alma Park Industrial Estate, Grantham, Lincs NG31 9SD
tel. 01476 541080; fax 01476 541061; orders@gbs.tbs-ltd.co.uk

North American agent/distributor: National Book Network
4501 Forbes Boulevard, Suite 200, Lanham, MD 20706;
tel. 301 459 3366; fax 301 429 5746; www.nbnbooks.com

Australian agent/distributor: Pan Macmillan Australia
Level 18, St Martins Tower, 31 Market St, Sydney, NSW 2000;
tel. 1300 135 113; fax 1300 135 103; customer.service@macmillan.com.au

New Zealand agent/distributor: David Bateman Ltd
30 Tarndale Grove, Off Bush Road, Albany, Auckland;
tel. (09) 415 7664; fax (09) 415 8892

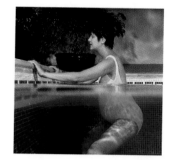

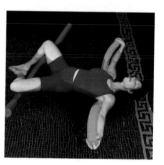

A CIP catalogue record for this book is available from the British Library.

Publisher: Joanna Lorenz
Project Editor: Debra Mayhew
Designer: Ruth Hope
Photographer: Christine Hanscomb
Production Controller: Darren Price

Previously published as Aqua Yoga

10 9 8 7 6 5 4 3 2 1

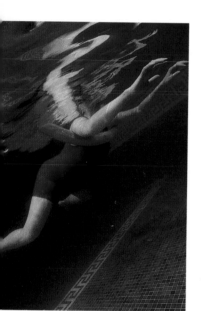

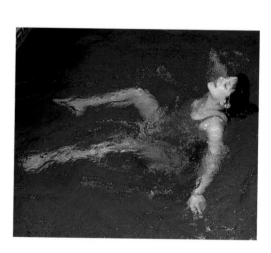

Contents

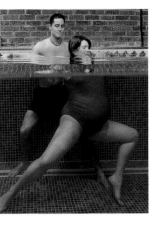

Forewords 6

section 1
Introducing Aqua Yoga 8

section 2
Antenatal Aqua Yoga 18

section 3
Antenatal Swimming 42

section 4
Antenatal Breathing & Relaxation 50

section 5
Preparing for a Waterbirth 58

section 6
Postnatal Aqua Yoga and Swimming 70

Water Relief Before and After Birth 92

Resources and Acknowledgements 94

Index 95

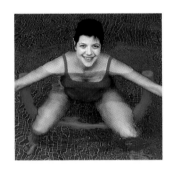

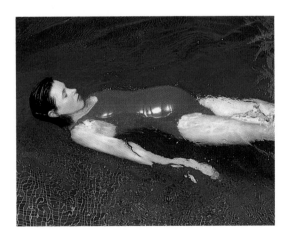

Forewords

IN RECENT YEARS there has been an increased awareness of the use of water during pregnancy, labour and delivery and the postnatal period. *Aqua Yoga* by Françoise Freedman provides an opportunity for parents to explore the benefits of promoting physical and mental wellbeing using water during the childbearing experience.

Aqua Yoga explores many ways of using water in preparing for birth, for delivery either in or out of water, and utilizes many years of experience to impart these skills to the reader. The power and supportive properties of water are discussed and the physiological and psychological benefits are shared by the author.

Françoise's book will add much to the quality of information available to parents wishing to use aqua yoga as a form of maternity care.

▽ For birth in
water, the non-
interventionist
approach allows
privacy, intimacy
and calm, whether
birthing at home
or in hospital.

Dianne Garland SRN RM ADM PGCEA MSC

Head of Maternity Services at Maidstone, Kent, Dianne Garland is also an advisor
to the Royal College of Midwives on waterbirth.

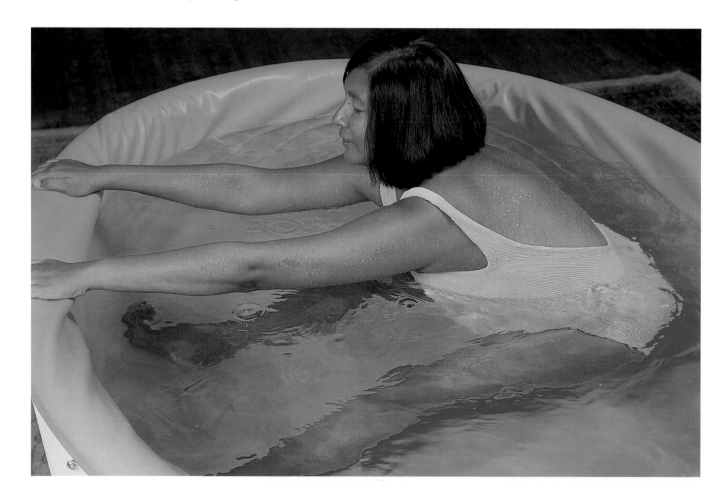

I USUALLY CLAIM that pregnant women should not read books about pregnancy and birth. Their time is too precious. They should, rather, watch the moon and sing to their baby in the womb. *Aqua Yoga* is an exception. As a mother of four and an anthropologist, Françoise has a deep-rooted understanding of the basic needs of pregnant women and of the relationship between human beings and water. This makes the content of her book safely and easily absorbed. This book is an ideal book for pregnant women.

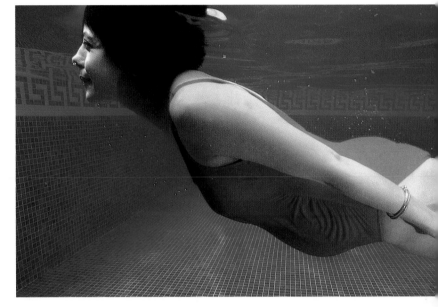

△ Aqua yoga revives the therapeutic power of water to ease childbirth.

It is during their pregnancies that many women develop an enhanced capacity to rediscover forgotten aspects of Human Nature. Via their strong attraction to water, many pregnant and labouring women tell us that Homo sapiens are more aquatic primates than is commonly believed. This makes sense in the current scientific context. It is difficult to imagine that after separating from the other chimpanzees our clever and curious ancestors did not take advantage of the high-quality food that is available in the estuaries and on the sea coasts. We should not forget that the bones of the famous "Lucy" were found in the sand among crab claws, and turtle and crocodile eggs.

Aqua Yoga offers also an unexpected opportunity to go back to the root of Yoga. As a means of stilling the human intellect, yoga originally consisted of exercises predominantly based on animal movements. I find it significant that Françoise repeatedly refers to animals adapted to water. The "water-boatwoman" exercise resembles the action of these insects on the surface of the ponds. The "water turtle" pose resembles a swimming water turtle and the term "dolphin dives" is highly suggestive. Let us add that swimming breaststroke is swimming like a frog and that crawling is a very archaic way to move.

We must pay tribute to Françoise for transmitting in such a clear and subtle way her understanding of Human Nature. She is the pioneer of a new style in childbirth education.

Michel Odent

Internationally famous childbirth pioneer, Michel Odent, is also the founder of the Primal Health Research Centre in London.

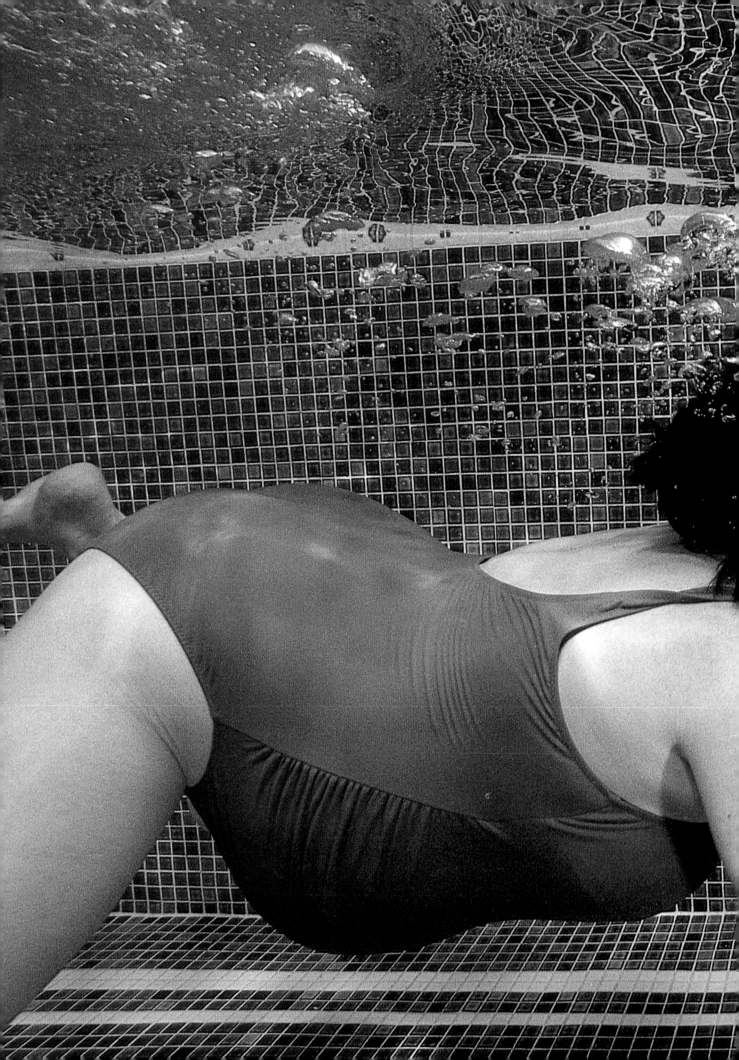

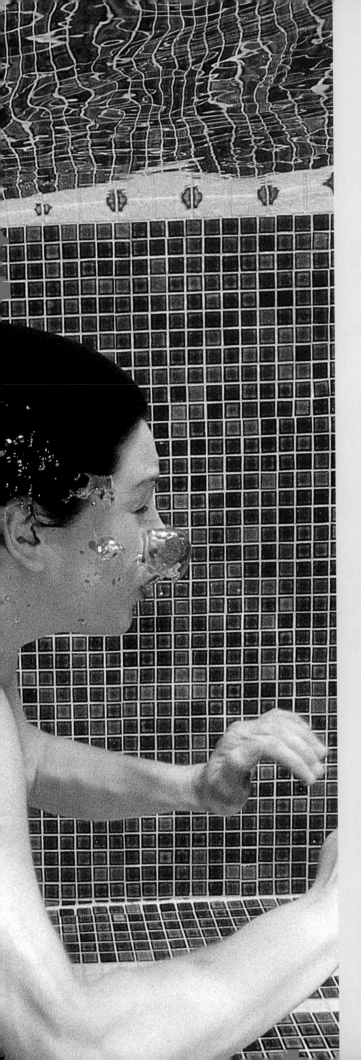

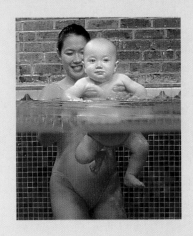

introducing
aqua yoga

Water is the source of life on this planet. It is an

environment familiar from before birth, as babies

grow in amniotic fluid. Water is an ideal medium

for yoga, allowing stretching and breathing beyond

anything that is possible in land-based postures.

The application of yoga to swimming increases

enjoyment and benefits, while floating relaxation

opens access to an anxiety-free state of harmony

with the surrounding world.

The benefits of aqua yoga

Aqua yoga is the most natural and all-encompassing way to promote and sustain fitness and health. It offers a gentle and easily available way to enjoy movement and breathing by using the supportive element of water. This book presents a combination of original exercises – many of them classic yoga postures adapted to water – with swimming strokes that have been found to be especially beneficial to mothers-to-be and new mothers, through experience, observation and many years of teaching.

Good health is far more than simply an absence of disease: vitality and contentment are required to enjoy pregnancy and the postnatal period fully. The power of water for revitalization and therapy has been known and used since ancient times by both humans and animals. The Greeks and Romans gave a high priority not only to baths but also to exercise in water. Massage in water can also be used therapeutically for healing injuries, as well as on specific areas of the body that need loosening, toning, strengthening and shaping.

Swimming for health

Swimming has been shown to strengthen the immune system, and can help to heal a wide variety of conditions. People with chronic illnesses, such as asthma, benefit

▷ **The supportive medium of water allows strain-free, ample movements of the hips while on your front …**

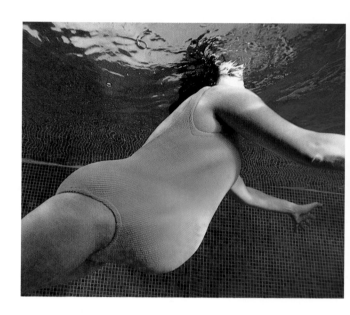

from its effects on their breathing, even finding that they shake off infections and other problems in no time at all. There are very few people who will not benefit from swimming and for whom it may be unsuitable. It is rated as the top exercise for stamina, suppleness and strength, as it exercises the whole body simultaneously, rather than working on parts of it separately.

Everyone can swim, regardless of their age or state of fitness. Supported by the water, joints and muscles can move freely, unhampered by gravity and protected from the jarring and knocking that can happen

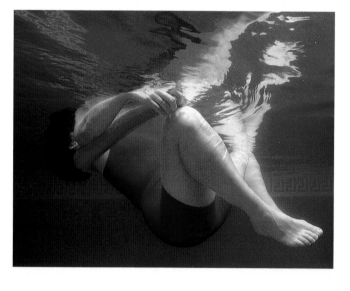

◁ **… and on your back, floating with a support if needed.**

in land-based exercise. It is ideal for all conditions, such as pregnancy, where weight-bearing exercise is best avoided.

The general benefits of swimming are well known. It increases lung capacity and improves breathing performance, increasing the tidal volume of the lungs as well as their blood supply. It also improves the proportion of muscle to fat, while strengthening the connective tissues (cartilages, ligaments and tendons), intermuscle and organ-supporting tissue. Lower-back problems and painful arthritic or inflamed joints can be alleviated by swimming.

Cardiovascular function and muscle tone are enhanced, and both the pulse rate and recovery period are reduced: this is really helpful during labour. The number of capillaries increases, as does the haemoglobin. Your recovery after surgery or from a weakened condition will be improved, which may be important if you have a traumatic birth or Caesarean section.

In summary, swimming not only improves the circulatory and respiratory systems but develops mobility in the muscles and joints and increases muscular strength and tone. Of all exercise forms, it performs these functions in a most effective and enjoyable way within a short time span.

Major skeletal muscles and ligaments for posture in pregnancy and after birth

Both in pregnancy and after birth it is extremely important to strengthen and elongate the muscles of the back, buttocks, thighs and abdomen. In aqua yoga, as in classical yoga, this is achieved through a combination of breathing and stretching, but greater elongation of muscle is possible in water.

Your deep spinal muscles, together with your leg muscles adjust your posture through pregnancy and after birth by holding your pelvis in the right position at all times, supporting your baby comfortably.

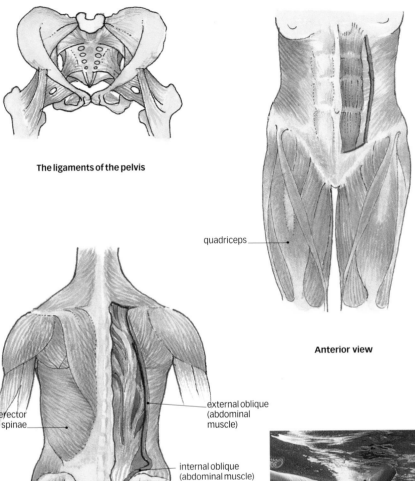

The ligaments of the pelvis

quadriceps

Anterior view

erector spinae

external oblique (abdominal muscle)

internal oblique (abdominal muscle)

buttock muscle

hamstrings

Posterior view

Breathing is what matters

Aqua yoga combines slow stretching with the use of breathing and relaxation, as the water provides resistance for the muscles to work against. Bodies feel virtually weightless in water, so that stretches that might not be possible on the ground can be achieved without strain. Although it is not yet practised widely, aqua yoga is a perfect combination of the benefits that yoga and swimming each can bring. Both share the practice of deep breathing. Swimming, involving exercise of the whole body with the deep breathing necessitated by its rhythmic movement, promotes the health of all tissues. Swimming that deepens breathing, stretches the body and calms the mind becomes the type of yoga described in the classic Indian texts.

This book is aimed at developing your fluidity. By cultivating a "go with the flow" attitude to life, you can simultaneously be active whilst surrendering to outside influences. Water is eminently supportive to yoga's pursuit of the essential inner balance, without which spiritual and physical harmony cannot exist. The time of creating a new life and bringing a child into the world, requires this unified harmony in a special way, and aqua yoga can uniquely respond to this.

▽ **Supported by water, the baby feels free and easy.**

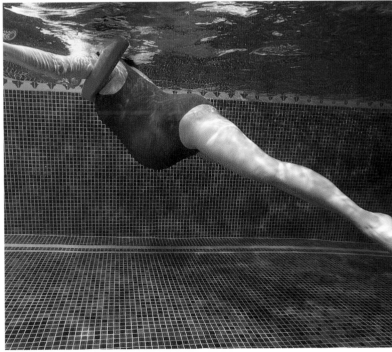

The essence of aqua yoga

The benefits of swimming, as a very efficient means of keeping the body in good condition and rapidly returning to fitness, apply well to women during pregnancy and after birth. It may be the only form of exercise that remains comfortable until the moment of birth.

In pregnancy, women do better if they exercise. The human body developed over many thousands of years in a harsh world, and it continues to need physical activity to stay in good order. Many of the common complaints of pregnancy are due to an inactive lifestyle. Aqua yoga makes it possible to get the exercise you need without undue strain or risks and in a relatively short time, achieving results with two half-hour sessions per week.

Both yoga and swimming are ideal forms of an overall fitness programme during pregnancy and postnatally, but aqua yoga is more than the sum of its parts. It will enhance your health and wellbeing while you are pregnant, and help to prepare both your body and your mind for birth.

Pregnancy requires special training of the body to respond effectively to the added

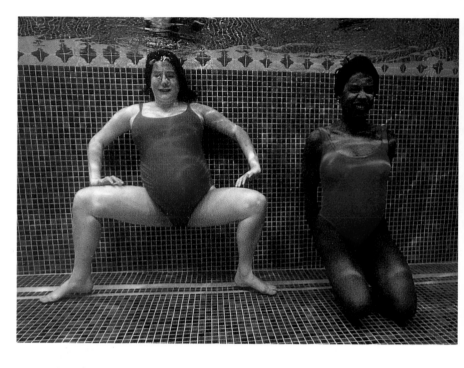

strains and stresses placed on it by weight increase and hormonal changes. If they are handled correctly, these changes can be experienced positively and greatly enjoyed during pregnancy and right through to the time when your baby is born.

△ Yoga helps you to open your body for birth, and then close it afterwards.

Exercising during pregnancy

A study in the United States showed that pregnant women who exercised in water had lower heart rates and blood pressure than women who did ordinary exercises. The babies also benefited by having lower foetal heart rates after water exercises than when the same exercises were done on land.

Because of buoyancy, water makes the body virtually weightless, so all pregnant women immediately feel more comfortable and free to move. The aches and pains in the lower back, neck and knees that are common in pregnancy, due to imbalance in the hips and poor posture, can be eased or cast off, and while you are in a horizontal swimming position your blood pressure is lowered and the risk of exhaustion from exercise is greatly diminished.

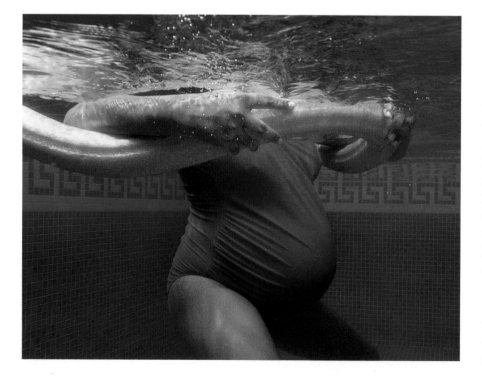

◁ In aqua yoga, the four layers of abdominal muscles are exercised effortlessly around the growing uterus.

Elongation

Aqua yoga promotes isokinetic contractions of the muscles as they are moved at constant speed in the water. This is better for women than exercise that tends to shorten muscles by developing tension through isotonic and isometric contractions.

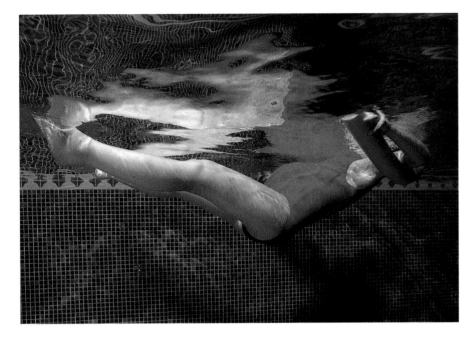

▷ Legs can be actively stretched in water right up until giving birth.

Aqua yoga combines the efficiency that both yoga and swimming confer on muscles in extracting oxygen from the blood and discharging waste products into the lymph. The uterus works most efficiently if it has a plentiful supply of richly oxygenated blood to wash away the toxins and carbon dioxide which build up with muscle action. Invigorating exercise improves your vitality and the tone of your body. It makes you feel attractive and fit and promotes sound sleep.

A strong heart

Aqua yoga is even better than yoga at increasing cardiovascular fitness without a decreased blood flow to the uterus. In water, body temperature is not raised during exercise, which is also beneficial to pregnant women.

Preparing for birth

Whether or not waterbirth is an option that you have chosen or that is open to you in the particular circumstances of your pregnancy, aqua yoga can be beneficial for you not only before the birth of your baby but also during your labour, when water can be your main source of pain relief.

Aqua yoga integrates the physical, emotional and spiritual. Pregnancy is always a time of intense changes and personal transformation, and aqua yoga can put your mind at peace. It facilitates relating to your baby in the womb and promotes powerful relaxation. It is good for the baby too, toning foetal muscles and inducing greater alertness long before birth.

The water facilitates the release of pent-up emotions that can create tension at the time of birth. Aqua yoga, even more than yoga, has direct effects on the nervous system, both calming and stimulating, which is needed for an ideal balance. It increases the occurrence of an optimal foetal positioning and presentation at birth, using pelvic rocks, rolls, swings and loops which are easier to achieve and therefore more effective in water.

It is also valuable postnatally to tone the muscles in depth around the newly contracted uterus, reshaping the figure and restoring health and firmness. So once you have given birth, return to the swimming pool – and why not involve your baby too?

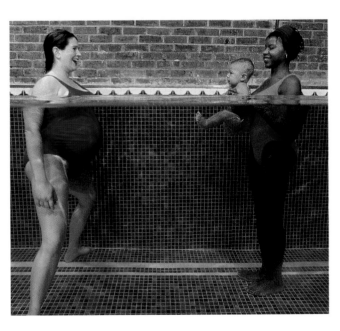

◁ From late pregnancy until the period following birth, yoga in water helps you keep your spine aligned in a sound posture.

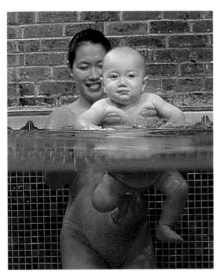

△ Your new baby is a welcome companion in postnatal aqua yoga.

Where and how to practise

You can do aqua yoga in the sea, in a river or a lake, but you are most likely to choose a swimming pool. The depth needs to be between waist and shoulder level: chest level is ideal. For aqua yoga swimming, a length of at least a few metres is needed, but for the aqua yoga sequences you will not need much more than the size of a yoga mat.

There may be several pools near where you live or you may have to make do with the only one within reach. In this case, it is better to adapt to a less than ideal pool than not to do aqua yoga at all.

Choosing a pool

Indoor heated pools are not affected by the weather and offer a guaranteed basic temperature and standard of sanitation. However there are many variables which can affect your enjoyment of aqua yoga, both antenatally and postnatally:

Water quality Most pools are still disinfected by chlorine, rather than ozone-treated.

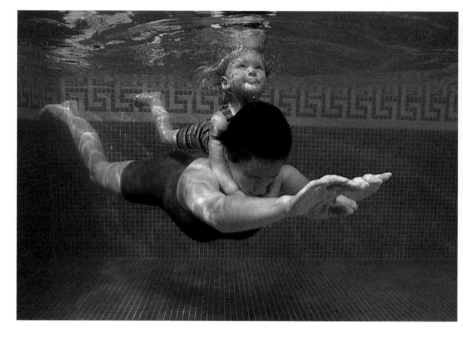

Chlorine may affect asthma sufferers and ozone is far preferable for young babies. Some pools are treated using a combination of ozone and sodium hypochloride; the latter acts as a residual disinfectant with fewer side

△ The practice of aqua yoga makes it easy to help your baby develop her natural swimming ability. She will enjoy accompanying you in the water through another pregnancy.

effects than chlorine. The overall standard of hygiene is important. Not only the water but the edges of the pool and the changing rooms should be clean and inviting.

Temperature The ideal temperature is 30°C/86°F. Training pools where children learn to swim are perfect for aqua yoga as they are usually slightly warmer than average, yet not as warm as some hydrotherapy pools, in which women in late pregnancy may feel too hot. If you wish to take your baby swimming, the pool needs to be as warm as possible.

Depth Training pools may be between 0.8m/2ft 7in and 1.45m/4ft 9in in depth throughout. Other pools may slope gently from a shallow end to a deep end.

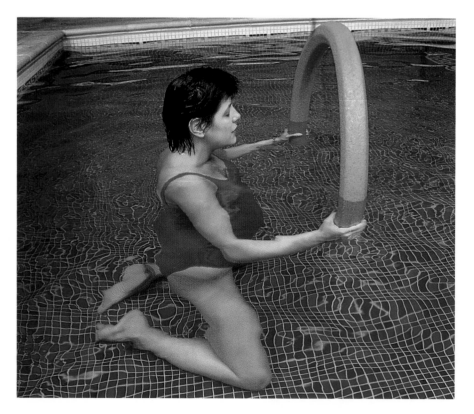

◁ A shallow pool is more comfortable to sit and kneel in, particularly for non-swimmers, but swimmers need to have access to deeper water.

Fixtures, access and safety Many training pools have bars which offer a steady support for hands and feet in the aqua yoga stretches. Other pools have a raised edge which can be used in the same way. Access into the pool may be by a ladder fixed to the side or by steps into the water. Steps are preferable to ladders in late pregnancy and if you are carrying your baby in and out of the pool. If there is no lifeguard in attendance, it is prudent to have someone with you at all times.

Size (for swimmers) Most modern pools are 25m/27yd in length, and training pools range from 8m/9yd to 12.5m/13½yd. Generally, a training pool is most suitable for aqua yoga. Doing lengths is fine if you are a confident swimmer, but forget about your ego and stay in the slow lane at least for your aqua yoga practice.

Convenience Take into account the distance you will have to travel, but seek out a well- managed pool. Many pools offer season tickets for regular swimmers and have special quiet slots in their timetables when you can stretch freely without being hemmed in by crowds. Some pools have times reserved for group bookings and it may prove cost-effective to arrange a weekly session with friends from your antenatal class or clinic.

Equipment for practice

Aqua yoga is a relatively cheap form of exercise, as very little equipment is needed. Buy a comfortable swimsuit that allows for

▷ Avoid dehydration. Drink while you are exercising in the pool if you need to, particularly if it is warm.

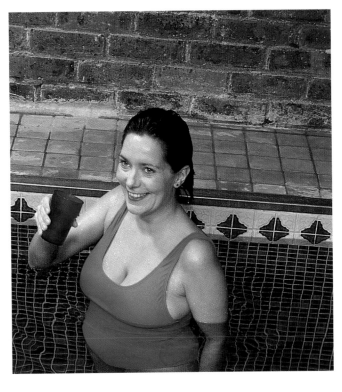

growth not only around your abdomen but also on the bust. Goggles will protect your eyes under water and provide clearer vision. Make sure they fit comfortably, particularly if you wear contact lenses.

Brightly coloured foam "woggles" (also known as "fun noodles" in the United States) are becoming an increasingly common sight at swimming pools and are ideal for supporting you during your aqua yoga sessions. If your local pool does not provide them, it is worth buying your own as they are fairly cheap. Refer to the end of this book for details of suppliers.

◁ Even if you are a good swimmer, it is worth investing in a pair of foam woggles (fun noodles) and a pair of floats that will give you full support to practise aqua breathing and relaxation. Some pools make these items available to swimmers on request.

How to practise

A session of 30–45 minutes is ideal. This will give you 10 minutes for exercises, 10 minutes for swimming and about 10 minutes for aqua breathing and floating relaxation. Always pay attention to the signals your body is giving you and stop when you feel you have had enough, which may be after only a few minutes in both early and late pregnancy.

Regularity is most important. It is better to visit the pool twice a week for half an hour than for one hour once a week. In late pregnancy, three short practices a week are most effective.

Besides observing general safety rules, take sensible precautions related to your pregnancy: be careful with temperature changes, rinse chlorine off your skin after swimming, allow more time to settle if you are driving home from the pool in late pregnancy. It is not advisable to swim if you have an infection, a rash, if you are bleeding or feel nauseous. Ask your midwife or doctor if you are uncertain about whether you should keep away from the pool and for how long.

Most important of all, make sure you are swimming for fun; this way you will get the most benefit from your practice. If you don't enjoy it, don't do it, but don't be deterred if you don't feel like swimming for a week, or a month, as hormonal changes can temporarily put you off. Try again later.

How to choose the best sequence

All the sequences presented in this book give equal importance to exercise, relaxation and the emotional preparation for birth. You may feel that you wish to concentrate specifically on one or more of these aims, and this is possible. Aqua yoga in pregnancy can be effective whether you are a keen swimmer or not and you will find variations to suit you whatever your ability, even if you do not usually enjoy the water. Do not be limited by preconceived ideas about your competence – just try it. Many women start tentatively, begin to enjoy it, and go on to improve their swimming skills after giving birth. All the antenatal sequences can be practised throughout pregnancy, indeed right up to the beginning of labour.

For maximum benefit, all the aqua yoga exercises follow the basic breathing pattern of yoga in which you inhale as you begin a stretch, extend fully on the beginning of your exhalation and release the stretch as you end your exhalation. Take your time to get used to this pattern, which may be unfamiliar to you, until you feel that it helps you find a very natural and effective rhythm. If you find this difficult, read the section on aqua breathing for a fuller explanation of how to use yoga breathing in water so that you familiarize yourself with it first of all.

Check your breathing at the beginning of each session, clearing both nostrils with Alternate Nostril Breathing (1). This will help to deepen your breathing before getting into the water. If necessary, learn to clear your nasal passages in water before getting into the pool. Fill a washbasin with water – salt water is best, so add some sea salt – then lower your face into the water and exhale sharply through your nose. You are now ready to begin your exercise, so enjoy!

Antenatal aqua yoga
The aims are:
- to enjoy a gravity-free environment
- to open the pelvis
- to stretch and strengthen the spinal and abdominal muscles
- to gain control of the pelvic floor muscles so that you can relax them while giving birth
- to expand your breathing capacity
- to relax more deeply and release worries and fears
- to "tune in" with your growing baby

About the antenatal exercises
The exercises are grouped into two main sequences. For the first, you are mainly standing in water, holding on to the bar or the edge of the pool, or to a foam woggle. This sequence is equally suited to swimmers and non-swimmers and, if you do not float, you can use supports for relaxing comfortably and safely in the water. The second sequence takes you away from the edge and involves more swimming skills, including adaptations of strokes combined with yoga stretches. For women who are both competent swimmers and familiar with yoga, some classic yoga postures are adapted for water. Each woman should choose her practice according to her ability and how she feels on the day: there are no "set" programmes to follow.

Both sequences involve going underwater, but you can also complete them without putting your face in the water if you dislike doing this. Going under water gives you greater freedom and helps to expand your breathing in a powerful way. Do not be limited by your perceptions of past experiences; many women find that these can be overcome as they go along. A good pair of goggles, and in some cases earplugs, may make being underwater more comfortable.

Some very good swimmers may prefer to swim lengths in their accustomed way rather than practise aqua yoga swimming.

1 Alternate nostril breathing
Two complete breaths form one round: do several rounds. Your breathing will deepen naturally, so you do not need to force it.

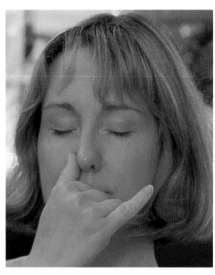

△ **1** Sit comfortably and erect. Bring your right hand in front of your face, with the three middle fingers tucked in towards your palm and the thumb and little finger extended. Place your thumb on your right nostril to close it, and breathe in through your left nostril.

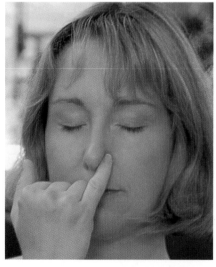

△ **2** Close the left nostril with your little finger and breathe out through the right nostril. Holding the hand position, breathe in through the right nostril, then close it with your thumb, open the left nostril by lifting your little finger and breathe out through it.

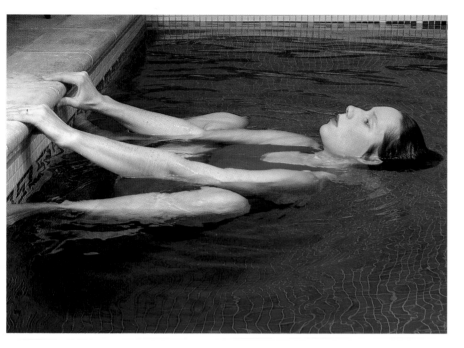

◁ The antenatal aqua yoga exercises activate the deeper muscles in the lower back and the pelvic area too.

each week. Some selection is needed so a few possible routines are suggested to start you off. Be careful not to overdo it and do not stay in the water for more than 45 minutes, particularly in late pregnancy. Ideally, include some standing exercises, some aqua yoga swimming and a relaxation each time. If you are not water-confident, make breathing your priority in the basic exercises so that you can feel your confidence increase at the same time as your buoyancy. Floating relaxation is also the foundation of supported swimming; this may gently but surely lead you on to unaided swimming.

After aqua yoga, you will be stimulated and your nasal passages will be clear. This is a good time to practise pranayama, the special breathing techniques of yoga, particularly if you have asthma or more general difficulty with breathing. A few minutes of Alternate Nostril Breathing (1) will again add greater benefit to your aqua yoga practice. You should always allow a few minutes of rest at the end of each session. As you may well be hungry after aqua yoga, it is nice to sit and enjoy a healthy snack at the pool rather than rushing out in a hurry.

▽ Relaxation is an essential part of your aqua yoga routine both before and after having a baby, particularly if this is your first child.

If practised well, swimming can only be beneficial. Yet the aqua yoga swimming sequence aims particularly at opening the pelvis and preparing the body for giving birth. It is useful to try the adaptations and the slow motion suggested, particularly in the third trimester of pregnancy, to get the full benefits of aqua yoga. Swimmers who do this find it helpful not only to prepare for the birth but also to refine their technique and expand their breathing.

If you intend to have a waterbirth, or to use water as pain relief during labour, this book will be helpful, especially the dedicated section. The earlier you start, the more effective aqua yoga will be to facilitate your labour and birth. If you are not a swimmer and dislike swimming pools, you can gain a great deal from practising the pelvic floor exercises, breathing and relaxation at home in your bathtub. Bathtime is popular with babies before they are born too.

Postnatal aqua yoga

The aims are:

- to realign the spine and strengthen the spinal muscles
- to tone and strengthen the abdominal muscles
- to regain full tone of the pelvic floor muscles
- to energize without strain in a short movement, relaxing at the same time
- to tone and remodel your figure safely
- to get ready to swim with your baby

About the postnatal exercises

Aqua yoga helps you close and tone your body again after giving birth, through sequences that mirror the antenatal ones. It is possible to start with these if you are reading this book and have already had your baby, though it may be helpful to look at the "opening" exercises in order to fully understand the reason for the "closing" ones.

Planning your practice

Start with the basic exercises (spinal alignment, pelvic floor and abdominal muscles, use of the breath) and progressively add on the other exercises when you feel ready, perhaps exploring two or three more

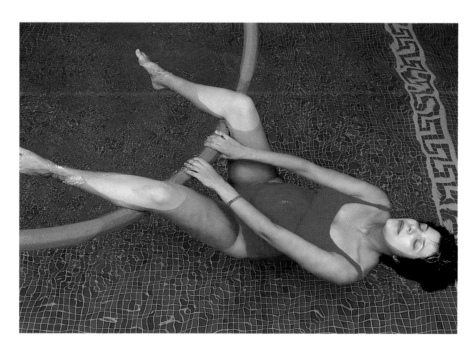

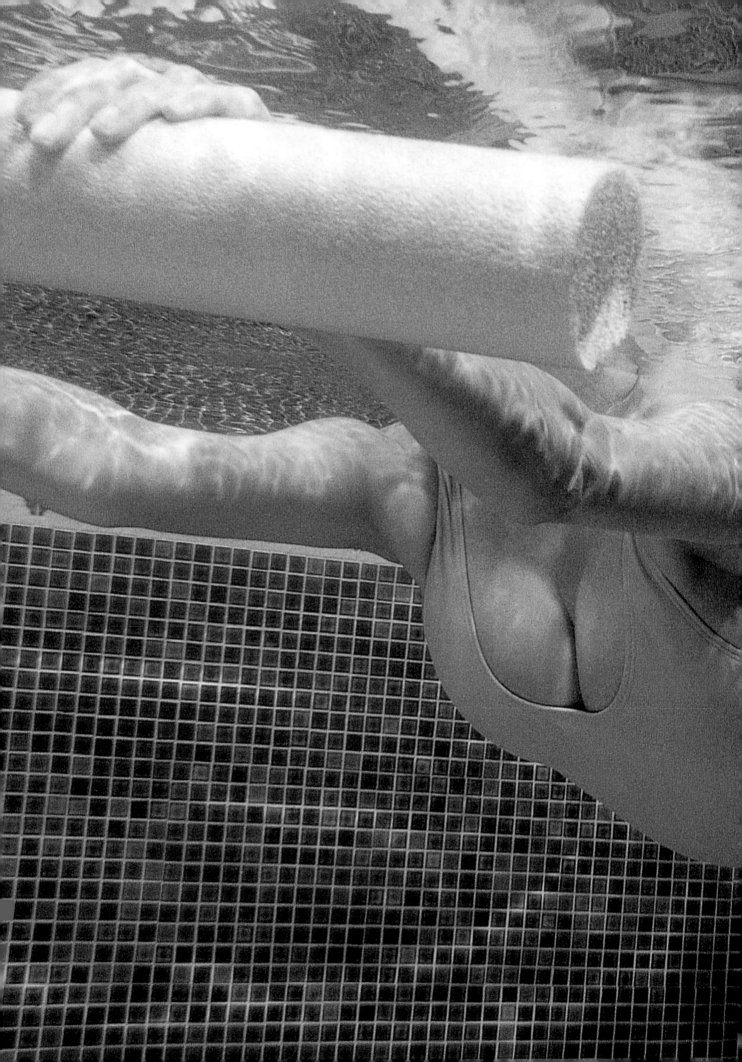

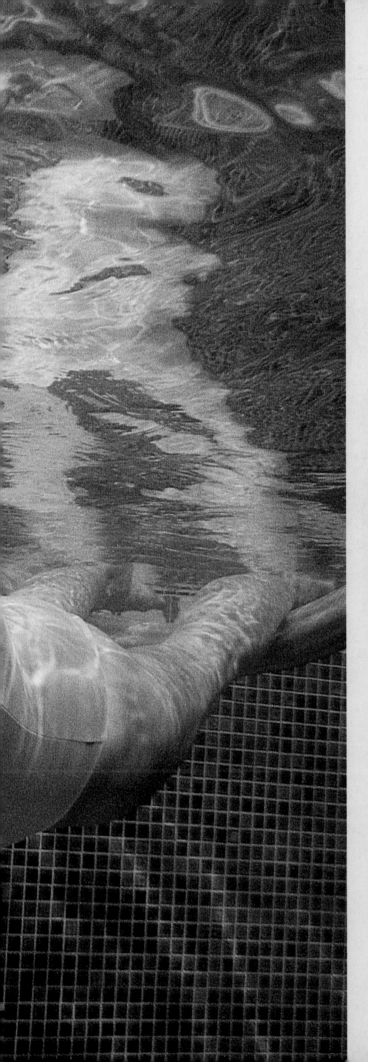

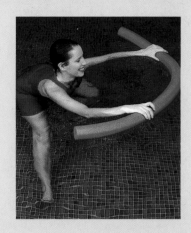

antenatal
aqua yoga

In pregnancy water gives freedom of movement.

It is a powerful toner and vitalizing medium.

In aqua yoga stretching, breathing and flowing

become one in water. The yoga exercises that

follow may look easy but are very effective in

toning and increasing the flexibility of pelvic

muscles. Water is an enjoyable medium in which

to approach birth in a vital, energized yet

profoundly relaxed way.

Aqua breathing

Breathing and relaxation in water are powerful tools to use for dealing with the emotional transformations of pregnancy. They create positive memories which the body can use efficiently in giving birth, and that babies may receive too. In the following exercises you are using not only your body but also your mind to control and expand your breathing in the water. Deeper, more expansive breathing has many benefits on the physiology as a whole and is of great importance in inducing confidence and calm. With practice, all the muscles of your pelvis become involved in your breathing, making it a powerful tool in labour.

2 Aqua breathing for non-swimmers

Find the position that is most comfortable for you to breathe. At the same time, in preparation for exhaling in long dives, feel the water as an environment that surrounds and supports you. Nose clips are not recommended as aids to learning how to breathe under water, because they can place additional pressure on the sinuses. It is better to get used to inhaling through the nose as you lift your face out of the water and exhaling through both the nose and mouth underwater.

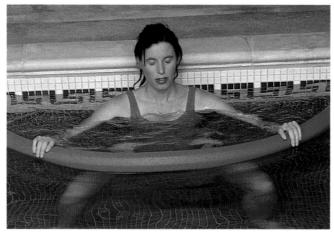

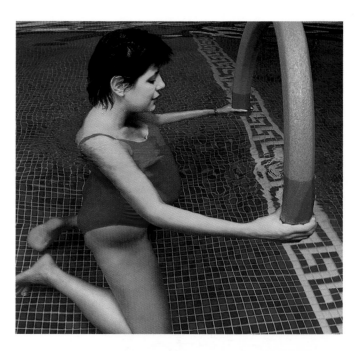

△ **1** You may like simply standing in the water, against the pool wall, with a woggle to support you.

▷ **2** If the water is not too deep you can kneel, leaning on a woggle or holding it to stabilize you.

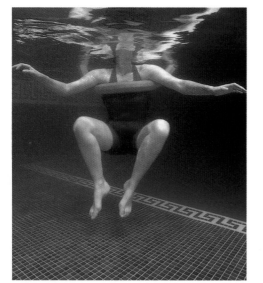

◁ **3** You can also float in an upright position, supported on a woggle.

▷ **4** Focusing on your breathing, extend your exhalation for twice the duration of your inhalation, counting to 2 when you inhale and 4 when you exhale, then to 3 and 6. Blow bubbles in the water if this makes it easier or more fun for you. You can also practise sinking to the bottom of the pool, which becomes increasingly difficult during pregnancy, slowly breathing out through your mouth.

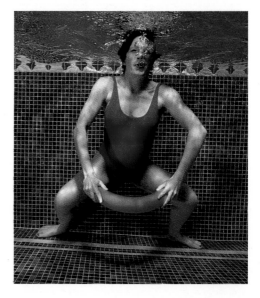

3 Supported breathing stretches

Two to four breathing stretches are a good preparation for floating relaxation at the end of your aqua yoga session. These stretches use floats or woggles for support. Try the different possibilities and choose the one which suits you best today. In a month's time your preferences and your skills may have changed. This exercise prepares you for the Breathing Dives with Relaxation (38) which is more comprehensive and effective.

If you dislike or cannot have your face in the water, inhale as you start and exhale as slowly as you can while you stretch forward without any movement of the arms or legs. The goal is to relax more and more as you reach the end of your forward movement and also the end of your out-breath. If you are able to put your face in the water, you will notice not only an increase in the forward movement but also a better combination of stretch and relaxation. You may like to chant or hum a tune as you are breathing out in your forward movement.

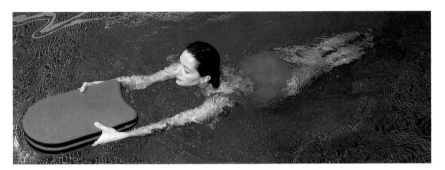

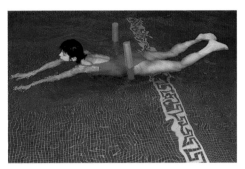

△ **1** Stand against the pool wall, holding a float or a woggle, and lower your body in the water. Pushing against the wall with your feet, knees bent, propel yourself forward with your arms extended, holding your float or woggle in front of you. You may find that your legs lower themselves in the water under you as you come to the end of your forward movement. Do not resist this, just relax as it happens and stand up when your feet touch the pool floor.

△ **2** You may prefer being supported by a woggle under your abdomen so that you can stretch your arms freely. You cannot be so streamlined as the woggle creates a transverse resistance, but your body can remain aligned until you run out of air in the stretch, without your legs going down.

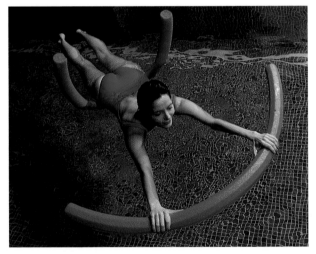

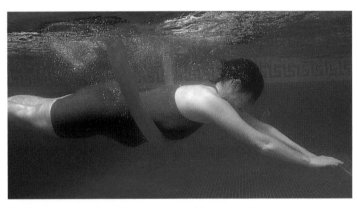

△ **4** If you are not a swimmer but you are reasonably water-confident and can go underwater, you can get the benefit of a dive with the support of a woggle under your abdomen. Inhale and push yourself gently off the wall to stretch, extending your arms forward and pointing them to the bottom of the pool in front of you. Blow out in the water and relax as you reach the end of your movement.

△ **3** For a fully supported stretch, use two woggles, one under the abdomen and the other in front of you so that you can hold it with outstretched arms.

4 Submerged breathing

If you are someone with a deep-seated, intrinsic fear of water, this exercise will be difficult at first, but most rewarding as you practise it.

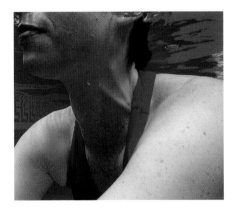

◁ **1** Extend your out-breath under water as long as you can, until you feel you have to reach out to fill your lungs again with fresh air. This stimulates your breathing overall and makes you feel the power of breathing. Do not stay under water after pressure builds up in your head. If you hear a ringing sound in your ears, lift your head out of the water and take a breath immediately.

Spinal alignment and awareness

As the uterus becomes heavier and its weight pulls on the ligament of the pelvis in the third trimester of pregnancy, the lumbar curve in the spine tends to become more pronounced. To compensate for this, as your body seeks to maintain its balance, the thoracic curve can also become exaggerated, which may produce "waddling" in late pregnancy.

Aqua yoga exercises prioritize the lengthening of the lower back and simultaneous toning of the pelvic ligaments and leg muscles, which together ensure the correct progressive adjustment of the pelvis throughout pregnancy.

The curvature of the spine in pregnancy
Your growing baby affects the curves of your spine.

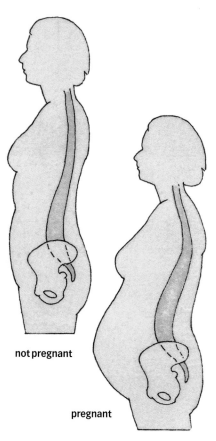

not pregnant

pregnant

5 Free standing in the water
Relaxed standing in the water at each stage of pregnancy will help with the mobility of the pelvis and free the lower back.

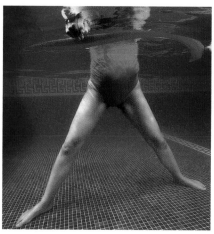

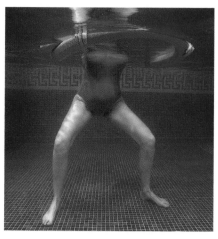

△ **1** Free standing can be done facing the wall and holding the bar or edge, or facing the pool using a woggle under the arms for support. Stand with your legs apart, aware of your straight spine and the muscles of the pelvic floor.

△ **2** Bend your knees, keeping your back straight, and lower yourself in the water with a sideways zigzagging movement down and then up. Then bend and straighten your legs and shake your arms loose. This "loop" helps you gain awareness of your spinal muscles while you let all the superficial muscles "wobble".

6 Drops
Easy to low squats will gently stretch the spine and are quite safe in the water. They allow women who are affected by pelvic pain to enjoy the benefits of easy squats with minimum risk and help them tone their pelvic ligaments.

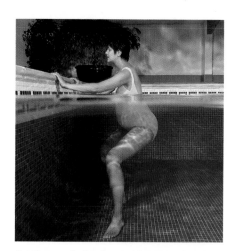

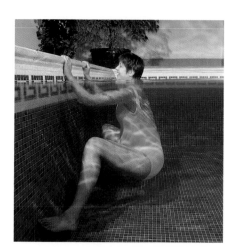

△ **1** First practise bending your knees outwards from a standing position with your legs apart, keeping your back straight. You can do this against the wall of the pool to help with alignment.

△ **2** As you flex your knees open, lower yourself in the water with a deep exhalation, keeping your back straight. Inhale as you return to a standing position. Do several small drops, lengthening the spine a little more each time.

Pelvic floor muscles

The pelvic floor, a deep "hammock" of muscles and fibrous tissues suspended between the coccyx at the back and the pubic bone at the front, supports your pelvic organs, the uterus, the bladder and part of the bowels. During pregnancy, both the increase in weight of the uterus and the hormonal softening of the muscles weaken the pelvic floor, particularly around the three openings of the urethra, vagina and anus and their respective sphincters. The Pelvic Floor Lift and Release (7), below, involves the deep muscles in the lower back and pelvis.

The muscles of the pelvic floor and perineum
As the main support of the uterus, the pelvic floor muscles need constant toning and strengthening.

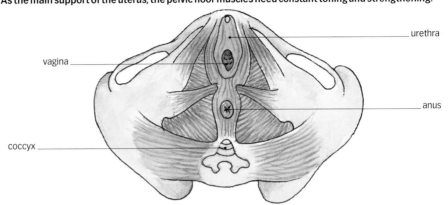

urethra

vagina

anus

coccyx

7 Pelvic floor lift and release

It is important to gain familiarity with your pelvic floor muscles, which support your uterus and must remain toned yet able to relax to allow your baby to be born without tearing or needing an episiotomy. In yoga, breathing and exercise are combined to obtain optimal tone in these muscles. These exercises are particularly effective in water, giving you a firm, supple pelvic floor and preparing you psychologically for the physical motions of giving birth. The best way to protect your perineum is to learn to relax it fully, which requires learning to contract it first. The two actions go together and, coupled with breathing, they reinforce each other. They also contribute to the maintenance of a healthy vaginal tone throughout pregnancy, an easier return to sexual intercourse after the birth, and long-term pelvic health.

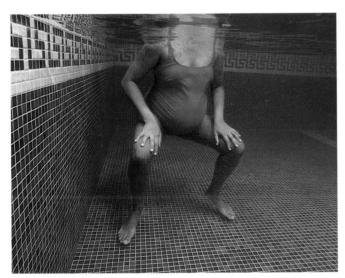

△ 1 Stand with your feet slightly apart. To locate your pelvic floor muscles, imagine that you are trying to stop yourself urinating in mid-flow (try this beforehand if necessary). Once you have found how to tighten the muscles, draw them in and up as you take a breath, involving your lower abdominal muscles as well. All this will become easier as you practise deep abdominal breathing in the water. Bend your knees outwards. As you breathe out, release all the muscles. Vocalizing your exhalation as "Aah" and making sure your lower jaw and neck are relaxed can help you feel this release even more. Repeat several times, concentrating on the feeling of the muscular action.

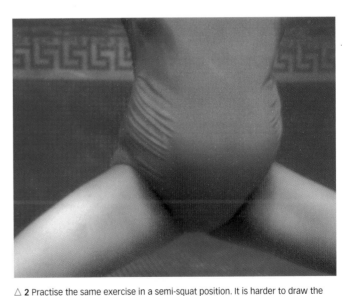

△ 2 Practise the same exercise in a semi-squat position. It is harder to draw the muscles up in this more open position, but also more powerful. You may find that you are also involving the muscles that hold the anus. These are useful when your baby is being born as as they are connected to your perineum and the birth is facilitated if they can be stretched and relaxed. With practice in this position you may come to feel separately the muscles that support the bladder. These are connected to the perineum at the front end, near your pubis.

Opening the body hip rolls and loops

Rolling and looping hip movements will help to open the hips while lengthening the spine and strengthening the knee and ankle joints. These ample movements are much easier in the water and can be done at all stages of pregnancy, helping to prevent or relieve backache. They will also help you to find your rhythm in movement in preparation for labour. Make sure you breathe rhythmically while doing the rolls and loops and enjoy the massaging action of the water on your body in these dynamic circling movements.

▷ **Before starting the rolls and loops, loosen your hips by bending one leg and then the other from a standing position with your legs wide apart, either against the wall or standing freely. If you are familiar with yoga, this is like the base of an Archer's pose in the water.**

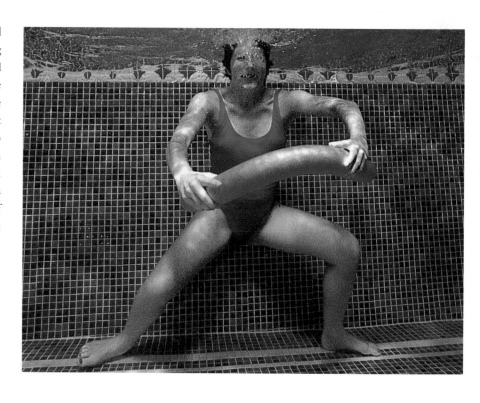

8 Hip rolls and figures-of-eight

Stand upright with your feet hip-width apart, supporting your hands and bent arms on the bar or pool edge. You can face the wall, which allows more traction in the loops, or face the pool, which helps you keep your back straight. Rolls relieve backache caused by uneven distribution of your weight, due to either your posture or the position of the baby, in mid to late pregnancy.

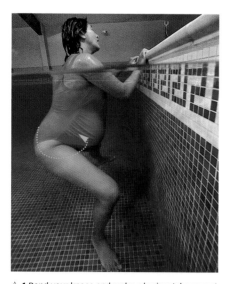

△ **1** Bend your knees and make a horizontal crescent movement with your hips from left and right. As you do so, find a good breathing rhythm that energizes you. Repeat the movement a few times, then extend the roll so that your hips are making a full circle. Circle your hips in both directions.

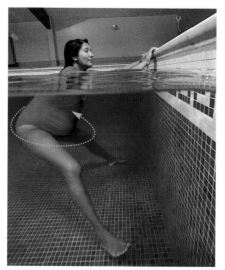

△ **2** Increase the intensity of the lower back stretch by opening your legs wider or extending your arms more to allow a wider circle. You can introduce a swing in the roll so that you are pulling more on the bar and bending your knees slightly further on the outer reaches of your circle.

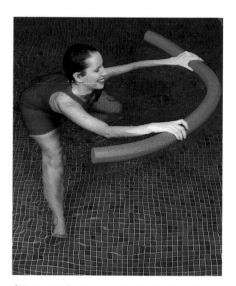

△ **3** You can also use a woggle to support you when doing hip rolls, which gives you more freedom but is a less energetic movement. To make a figure-of-eight roll your hips from left front to right back and from right front to left back in a continuous curving motion that stretches your whole spine as you go.

9 Hip loop forward and back

You can make this sinuous loop as small or as extreme as you wish. If you feel very energetic, you can make it more dynamic by positioning your feet wide apart and looping into a low squat. Paradoxically it may feel easiest to do this when you are in late pregnancy. Keep your head relaxed and be aware of the alignment of your spine throughout: your legs and arms are the bending stretchers in this exercise while your spinal and abdominal muscles are stretched and toned.

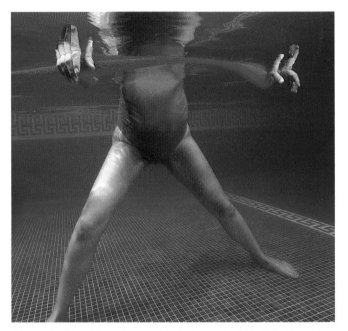

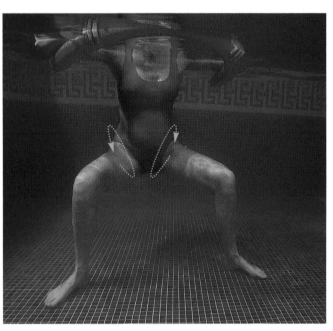

△ 1 Stand upright with your feet apart, facing the pool wall, ideally holding on to a bar if there is one, or onto a woggle. Keeping your arms bent, inhale, bend your knees and let yourself drop as you exhale.

△ 2 Thrust your pelvis forward and straighten your legs as you come up, then, with your back extended, lean your trunk forward and bend your knees again to roll forward. Continue the movement as a loop, forward and back. You can then reverse the loop.

10 Hip wheel

For the standing exercise, it does not matter whether you are facing the wall or the pool. Support your hands, with bent arms, on the bar, pool edge or a woggle. You can make the exercise more dynamic by having your feet further apart and therefore widening the wheel. You can also go into a deeper squat on the way down. Most of all, make sure you adopt a comfortable starting position that allows you to enjoy this hip wheel.

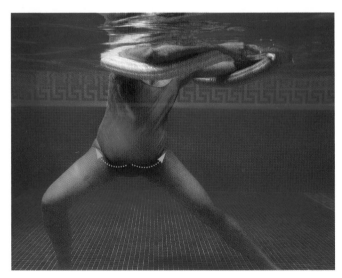

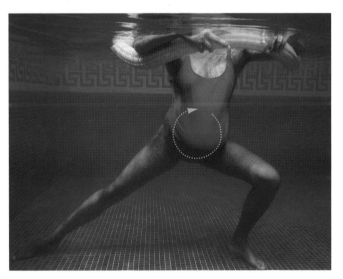

△ 1 Begin with your feet wide apart. Bend your knees and swing your pelvis slowly from side to side in a vertical crescent, keeping your back very straight, finding a good breathing rhythm as you go down and then up.

△ 2 When you are comfortable with this swing, take your hips all the way round and make a wheel, going down again on the other side, bending your knees as you go down, straightening them as you go up in a smooth, rhythmical movement, inhaling as you go up and exhaling as you go down.

Hip openers

Once you have loosened your lower back with rhythmical rolls and loops, you can proceed to further stretching of the ligaments and muscles in the pelvis, particularly those that control the hip movements. The hormones progesterone and relaxin that are produced in your pregnant body give you greater flexibility in your joints. This makes it possible to overstretch dangerously on dry land, but the risk is eliminated in water. Conversely, if you are normally stiff, water can help you increase your flexibility.

11 Opening steps

Stand upright in the pool, facing the wall or the pool and with your hands on the bar or pool edge. Keep your arms slightly bent. You can also support your arms on a woggle, facing the woggle or with your back to it. If you are facing the wall, you can wedge your feet at the base of the wall on the pool floor while doing ankle rotations, which may help to prevent swelling in late pregnancy.

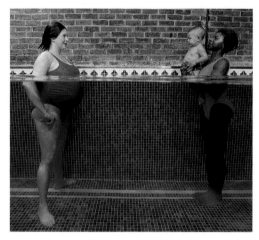

△ **1** Stand with your feet apart, keeping your legs straight. Turn one foot out and rotate the ankle outwards in small circles. Extend your toes to the pool floor as your foot stretches fully in the circling movement. Repeat with the other foot. In late pregnancy, hold on to the side of the pool for balance or place your hands on a woggle in front of you.

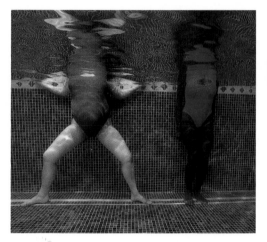

△ **2** To increase the stretch, open your legs slightly wider and bend your knees, turning your feet out. You can also turn one foot in and one foot out at a time, moving sideways in steps that open your hips. There is something funny about this exercise, so enjoy it. Make sure you keep your upper body relaxed all the time as you bend down.

12 Russian squats

You may be surprised at being able to do this exercise in water while you could not contemplate it on dry land even if you were not pregnant! It allows a deep squat while keeping your spine straight. During late pregnancy, both Russian squats and the open stretch that follows help the baby's head to engage in the pelvic outlet at the best possible angle, while you make the greatest possible use of gravity in preparation for labour. In a shallow pool, Russian squats can be practised from a kneeling position, with a short squat in-between as you change legs.

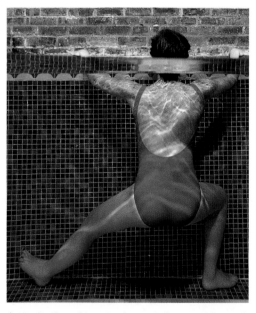

△ **1** Facing the wall or supporting yourself on a woggle, stand upright and let yourself drop in the water, keeping one leg bent while stretching the other into your heel in the fashion of Russian folk dancing. Keep your shoulders straight and your hips forward to elongate your spine.

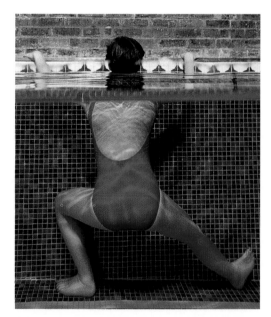

△ **2** Jump up as you change legs so that you stretch alternate sides in a vigorous rhythm, keeping your back upright throughout the movement, lowering the base of your spine.

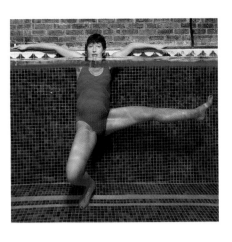

◁ **3** Once you have gained some experience stretching your leg with your heel on the floor, you can try to stretch it higher in the water. It is more strenuous, but your bent standing leg allows you to keep your back straight throughout the exercise, which is easier against the wall.

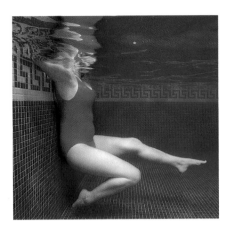

◁ **4** A variation of this exercise is to lift your leg straight in front of you in the water and bring it down bent, changing legs with a little jump. The resistance of the water makes this a more strenuous movement than it may seem at first sight.

13 Open stretch and pelvic swing

For the open stretch you can face the wall or the pool, or use a woggle for support. The pelvic swing can only be done using a bar to support you. It is a very helpful exercise to prepare for the letting go that is required at the second stage of labour, when the head of the baby is ready to be born.

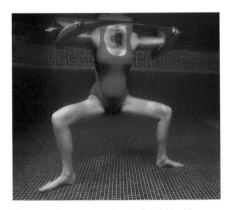

△ **1** To do the open stretch, stand upright with your arms bent and your whole body relaxed, and let yourself drop on an exhalation while opening your bent legs wide. If you are facing the wall, it can help to wedge your feet against the base of it.

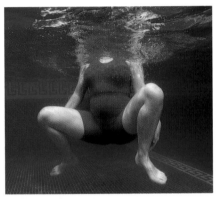

△ **2** To make this stretch even more open, drop further down, opening your bent legs wider. Breathe as deeply as possible while you stretch. Repeat several times, letting yourself drop slowly, stretching wide and coming back to the centre to a standing position between drops.

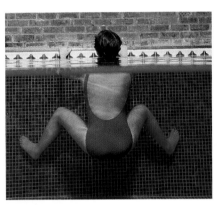

△ **3** For the pelvic swing, lower yourself in the water facing the wall and holding on to the bar, with your hands shoulder-width apart. Open your legs wide and bring them up so that you can wedge your feet on the pool wall with your knees slightly bent. Swing your pelvis back so that both your legs and arms stretch out, and then forward again close to the wall.

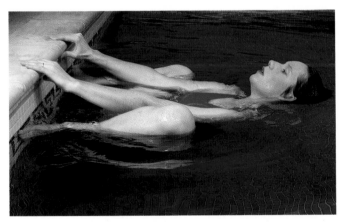

△ **4** To increase the stretch, bring your perineum as close to the water's surface as possible and swing further back. Find a rhythm that suits you and breathe as deeply as possible in a broad swing. The pelvic swing can be combined with a pelvic floor muscle exercise. Inhale and lift your pelvic floor muscles as you swing backwards and release them as you exhale in the forward swing.

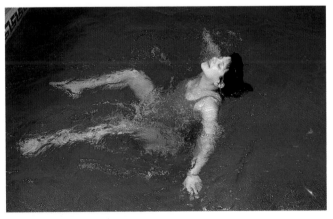

△ **5** You can also do a pelvic swing using a woggle for support, either in front of you or behind you. Focus on your pelvic floor, exhaling and releasing all tension in a slow forward movement of the hips.

Kneel open and swing

For these exercises, kneel down on the floor of the pool or, if the water is too deep for this, hang down from a support – the bar or a woggle – with your knees open and your legs loose. After stretching the base of the spine and opening the lower back with the hip openers, you are now stretching the muscles in the front of the body, particularly all the abdominal muscles. These exercises are toners for the thigh muscles as well as helping you to expand your abdominal breathing. The stretching of the lower back and abdominal muscles is combined in rhythmical movements, circling forward and back.

14 Kneel down and turn

The closer to the wall that you are kneeling in this exercise, the greater the stretch will be and the straighter your back. It is also an ideal way to practise your pelvic floor lifts, drawing in your muscles as you inhale and relaxing them as you exhale.

▷ **1** Holding the edge of the pool or a woggle, lower your knees wide open as far as you can, letting them rest on the pool floor if the depth of the water allows it. Breathe as deeply as possible in the whole abdominal area up to the diaphragm, keeping relaxed.

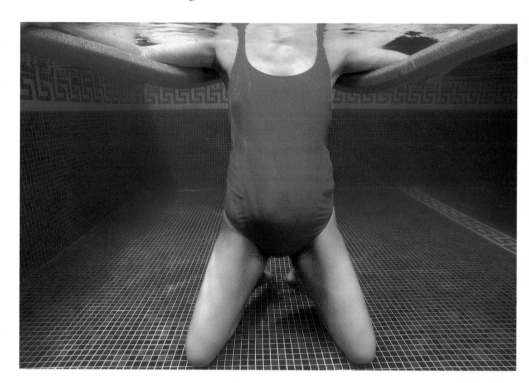

▷ **2** Lift one knee up and turn it out while placing your foot on the pool floor, opening the hip on that side. Keep your knee as straight above your foot as possible. Alternate right and left turns in a rhythm that suits you, taking time to breathe deeply and stretch fully.

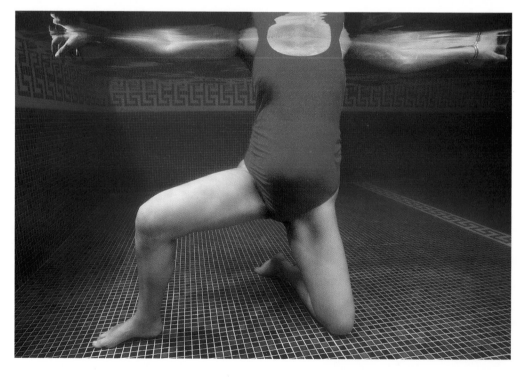

15 Kneeling archer pose

You can achieve this classic yoga pose even if you are new to yoga. It tones your buttocks and thighs and energizes you as you breathe in. If your pool is too deep to practise the kneeling pose, go directly to the standing archer pose.

▷ **1** Begin in the kneeling position from the previous exercise, with one knee turned out. Keep your trunk upright as you turn your raised knee out and breathe into the stretch that is created. Repeat on the other side.

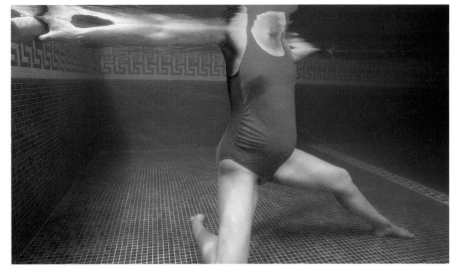

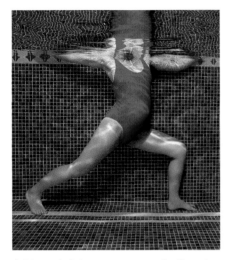

△ **2** As you feel stronger, you can practise the archer pose. Stand with your back to the pool wall and your legs wide apart. Bend one leg and turn out your hips and torso to face your front knee. Keep your back leg extended. Breathe deeply into the leg stretch. Your front knee should be directly above your foot. If you are experienced in yoga, you may be able to keep your back foot flat on the pool floor, but do not worry if your heel comes up to allow your hips to turn.

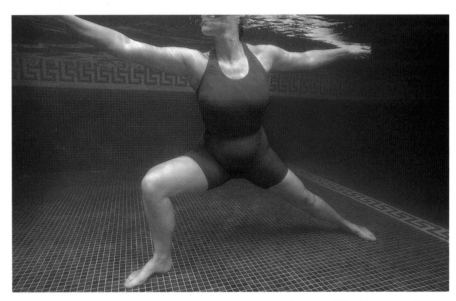

△ **3** As well as being done along the pool wall or holding a woggle to gain more stability, this pose can also be done free-standing in the pool, and in its full version it involves an extreme stretch. On your firm base, take a deep inhalation and extend both arms equally. Exhale in this stretch and breathe two more times as deeply as you can from the lower abdomen before bringing your arms down. Repeat on the other side.

16 Swing from kneeling to squatting and back again

This exercise can be done either facing the wall or the pool and holding on to the bar or edge, or using a woggle as a support. This is a grounding, opening exercise that can be practised throughout pregnancy and facilitates an optimal position for your baby as birth approaches.

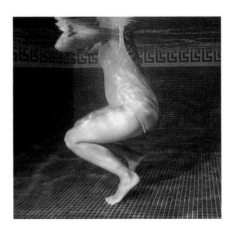

◁ **1** Start by kneeling on the pool floor with your knees wide open, breathing deeply. Lower your spine and lift both knees at the same time, bringing your legs forward into a squat. Hold for a moment, then lower your knees again to go back to a kneeling position.

▷ **2** At first you can shift from kneeling to squatting very slowly. Once you are familiar with the exercise, you can do it in a dynamic fashion, jumping from kneeling into a squat and back into kneeling, inhaling as you jump and exhaling as you reach the kneeling and squatting positions.

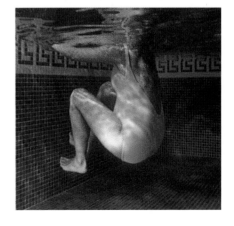

Knee and hip circles

In these exercises one leg is raised to rotate and open the hip, involving all the lower back muscles on that side as well as the pelvic muscles. They both prevent and relieve lower back ache and more particularly sciatica or inflammation due to the carrying of weights. If you have backache at any time during your pregnancy, focus on this sequence. Start with the small knee circles before proceeding to the wider hip circles and do them very slowly, with your leg moving as much water as possible.

17 Knee circles

For this exercise, face the wall and hold on to the bar or edge of the pool. You can also rest your arms on a woggle in front of you. The same exercise can be done facing the pool and supporting yourself on the bar or edge from behind, or on a woggle under your arms and behind your back. While facing the wall, the main stretch is in the lower back; facing the pool a greater emphasis is placed on opening the pelvis. This is a timely exercise to practise when you feel the stretching of your pelvic ligaments, sometimes painfully, as you reach the fourth to fifth month of your first pregnancy.

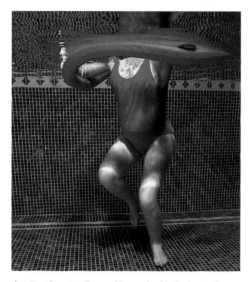

△ **1** Start in a standing position and, with the knee of your standing leg slightly bent, lift your other leg bent from the pool floor. Keep your upper body relaxed.

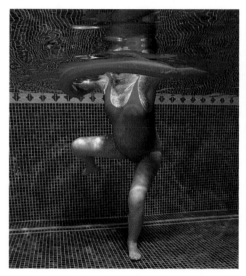

△ **2** Make small smooth circles with your knee in the water, keeping your whole body relaxed and feeling the resistance of the water. Repeat, changing legs.

18 Hip circles

Start in a standing position, facing the wall and holding on to the bar or the edge of the pool, or resting your arms on a woggle in front of you. Keep your standing leg a little more bent than for the knee circles, to allow for a wider opening of your other leg as you engage your hip in the rotating movement.

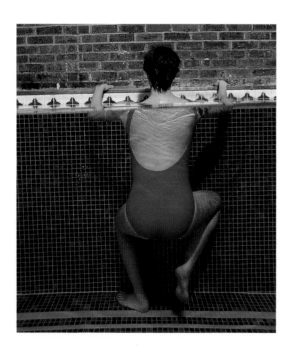

◁ **1** Circle one leg and hip several times slowly, keeping the knee bent and feeling the resistance of the water.

▷ **2** Make small circles at first and, as you become stronger, push your raised knee as far back as possible to increase the stretch. Breathe deeply exhaling each time you open out your knee. Repeat on the other side.

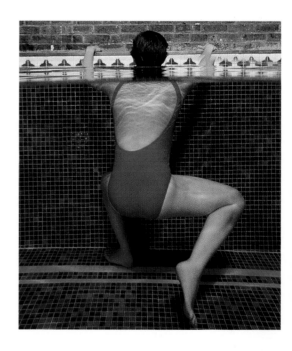

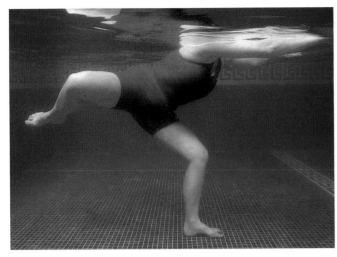

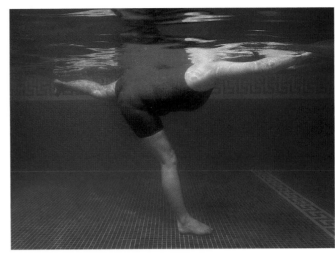

△ **3** Instead of circling with your leg bent, extend it and stretch it behind you, bending it again to come back to the centre. Breathe as fully as possible, using your abdominal muscles.

△ **4** After a few circles, you can extend your raised leg back behind you before bringing it back to a standing position. As you become fitter, extend your leg higher towards the surface of the water, straightening your standing leg.

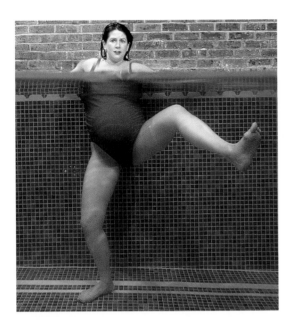

◁ **5** The hip circles can also be practised facing the pool or supporting yourself with a woggle behind you. They open the hips wide on each side while enabling you to keep your back straight against the wall or with the woggle.

▷ **6** Supporting your extended arms on the bar, pool edge or woggle, circle both hips with a wide backstroke movement of your legs.

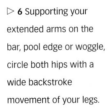

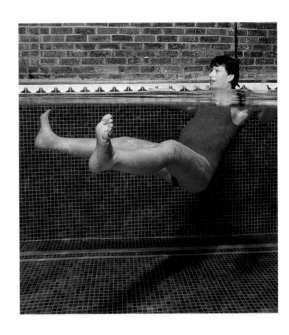

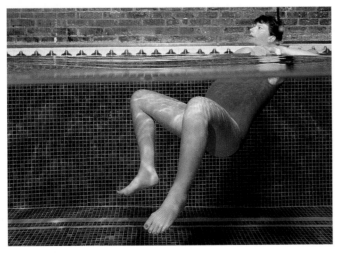

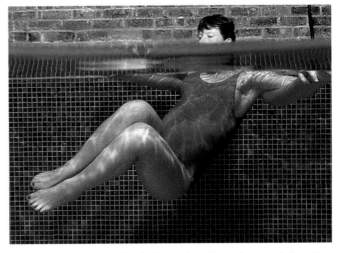

△ **7** Inhale as you stretch out, exhale as you bend your legs in. Keep the upper part of your body as relaxed as possible.

△ **8** Complete the circling with a double rotation. With practice, your circling will become smoother and more regular. If you are not a swimmer, include this exercise in each of your aqua yoga sessions during pregnancy as it is a good substitute for swimming on your back.

Arms and shoulders

These exercises make use of the resistance of the water to tone the muscles of the upper body. During pregnancy, you may find that the outer part of your upper arms, like your thighs, are areas in which body fat may accumulate. Regular exercise will keep this to a healthy minimum and your arms will stay shapely. Aqua yoga tones the muscles that support your breasts through a combination of held postures and rhythmical movements. Moving your arms under water is more energetic than it looks and strengthens your heart, which is essential to an active, healthy pregnancy. These exercises are designed to be a gradual and gentle training of your chest muscles to help your heart work harder as your baby grows, so that it can cope with the exertion of labour without reacting wildly. You can do them at your own pace, without strain, whatever your level of water skills. In a few minutes of moving your arms vigorously in water, you will not only feel stimulated but may wonder what was worrying you before you got into the pool.

19 Water sun wheels

A graceful but very intense exercise that tones all the back muscles as well as the arms and shoulders.

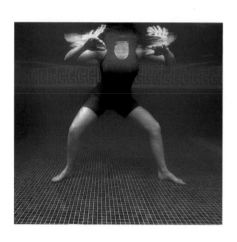

◁ **1** Standing in the water, bend your knees so that the water comes up to your neck. Move your arms forward and back, making figures-of-eight in the water, then open your arms and cross them in front of you with a sculling movement of your hands.

▷ **2** Extend your arms down in the water and stretch them outwards, pushing the water away from your body. Come back to the centre and repeat the movement, pushing away slightly higher towards the water's surface each time. Breathe deeply into the rhythm of the movement.

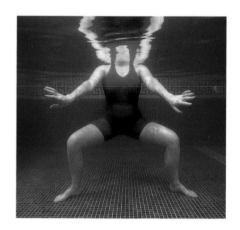

20 Arm twists

While your hips and legs make an open base, these two arm twists tone your upper back muscles and open your chest. The more your arms are immersed below the surface of the water, the more effective the exercise will be. The second arm twist is asymmetrical and makes use of an energetic rhythm in the stretch.

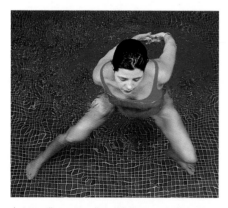

△ **1** Kneeling or standing with legs open wide and bent in the pool according to depth, clasp your hands behind your back, turning your shoulders out. Pull on your arms as much as possible, while breathing deeply, to move your shoulders right and left with an intense stretch in the pectoral muscles as well.

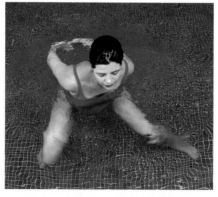

△ **2** If you are in a half-squat standing position, you may find it helpful to bend your legs alternately on each side as you stretch.

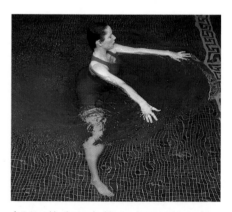

△ **3** Stand in the pool with your legs apart to make a strong base, bending your knees if necessary so that your arms can stretch in front of you just below the surface of the water.

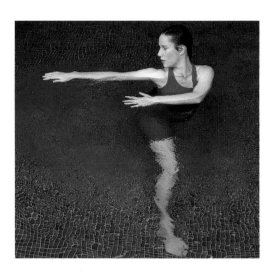

◁ **4** Inhale and swing your shoulders to one side, stretching the arm on that side and letting the other one follow the movement in a relaxed way as you exhale. Allow your head to follow the spinal twist rather than to lead the movement.

▷ **5** Inhale and turn to the other side in a swinging movement. Your knee on the stretching side will tend to bend, increasing the movement on a stable base.

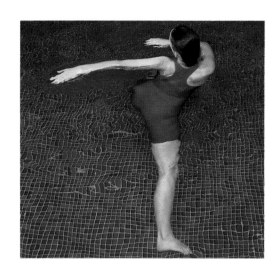

21 Standing and supported breaststroke

The arm movement of breaststroke opens the chest and stretches the upper back and arms in a way that is ideal throughout your pregnancy. Even if you cannot swim breaststroke, practising the arm movement as an exercise has its own merit. It can prevent and cure heartburn in early and late pregnancy, as well as gradually making more space for the growing baby under the ribcage. It is also a good exercise to keep your breasts naturally supported as they grow larger and heavier. Three different versions are presented here.

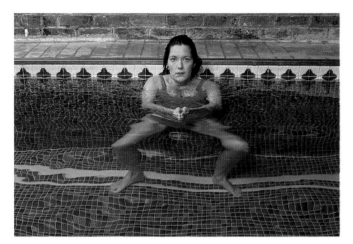

△ **1** Stand with your knees slightly bent if necessary so that the water comes up to your neck, or kneel if the water is shallow. Stretch your arms together in front of you, with the palms of your hands facing each other.

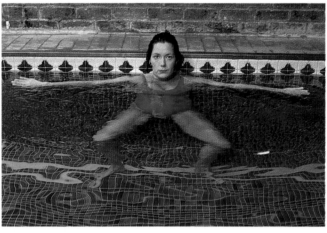

△ **2** Turn your hands out and open your arms in a wide circling movement, going as far back as possible before returning to stretch your arms again, and repeating the movement several times in your own rhythm. Inhale open, exhale back.

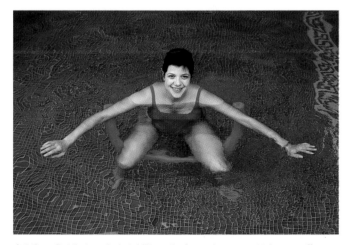

△ **3** If you find that you lack stability as the forward movement takes you off your base, you may want to use a woggle under your knees and stand in a semi-squat in the pool. This will give you a wide, supported base when stretching your arms.

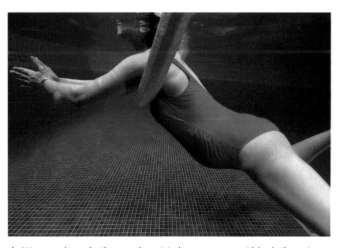

△ **4** You can also make the same breaststroke arm movement lying in the water on your front supported by a woggle. Keeping your legs and head relaxed, repeat the arm motion described in step 1. Breathe in as you extend your arms.

Aqua yoga poses

On dry land, stretching in yoga is achieved against gravity in standing, sitting and kneeling, prone and supine poses called "asanas" which, together with deep breathing, are the hallmark of yoga as a unique form of exercise. Water allows a greater freedom of movement and facilitates relaxation in the stretch itself. While in theory most yoga poses can be adapted to be practised in water, some lend themselves to aquatic versions better than others.

During pregnancy, poses that open the hips and stretch the whole body are particularly valuable. Three classic asanas are presented here in their aquatic versions, and can be practised throughout pregnancy. Since only a small proportion of pregnant women can float, relax and stretch at the same time, you will probably need to use a supporting woggle or foam board to align your spine in the stretch and get the maximum benefit from floating poses.

Take your time to get into each of these three poses and enjoy them as you breathe fully in the stretch. If you are a swimmer, what is asked from the body here may be quite new to you. If you practised yoga before you were pregnant, the aquatic adaptation of these three poses may help you adapt other asanas which you particularly enjoy on dry land, first in standing and then in floating versions. Start from bent knees to enjoy a fuller stretch.

22 Warrior balance

Although warrior poses and water may seem contradictory, the aquatic versions offer a strengthening and energizing stretch just like the land-based classic postures. Water facilitates a sound grounding at the bottom of the pool without strain. Rather than raising the arms up, they are extended on the surface of the water, to allow an intense stretching of the inner leg muscles in the balance that follows the warrior pose taking off to float forward.

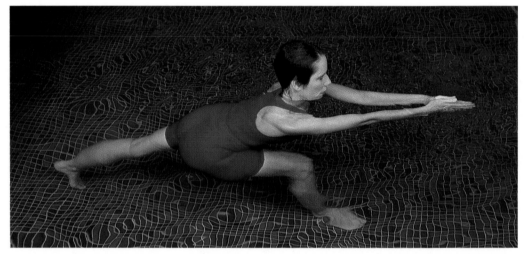

△ **1** Stand in the pool, inhale and take a wide step forward, bending your front leg so that your knee is above your heel and keeping your back leg extended, front foot solidly on the pool floor and turning out slightly to open the hips. Extend your arms in front of you, palms facing each other, and feel an intense stretch on the side of your back leg as you exhale. Even if you already practise yoga, it may be difficult to keep your back heel on the pool floor. Stretch from the base of your toes, extending the back of your knees. Take a few breaths in this pose, finding more extension in your middle back with each exhalation.

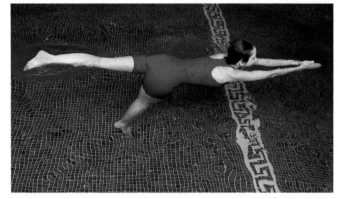

△ **2** While you inhale, stretch your front leg as you shift your weight forward on to it and raise your back leg slowly into a balance as you exhale. The buoyancy of the water transforms this balance instantly into a long relaxed floating stretch, as your body extends forward with the movement and the two legs join together.

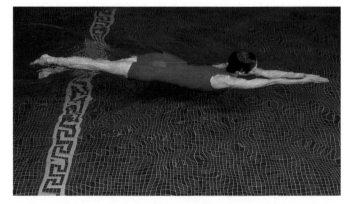

△ **3** Your body is now streamlined from the toes to the fingertips. Repeat this balance with the other leg and practise it a few times until you become familiar with the coordination of the movement and the breathing.(You may hold a foam board in the pose to achieve a full floating stretch at first.)

23 Floating tree pose

The tree pose is a classic yoga posture. One leg is bent, with the foot resting on the inside of the other leg in order to achieve an energizing yet calming alignment of the whole body. The arms extend over the head and ideally the hands are joined, palms facing each other, while the head remains in line with the spine. The aquatic version of this pose is best done with the support of a woggle or foam board in pregnancy, to allow a perfect alignment of the hips with the shoulders and legs in the water. A woggle or board under the base of the buttocks helps stabilize the pose, which only very good swimmers who practise yoga might sustain without support. In this pose, you stretch, relax and breathe deeply all in one. Two alternative ways of getting into the pose are presented.

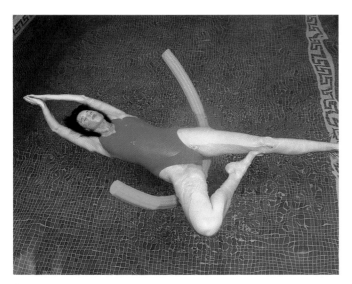

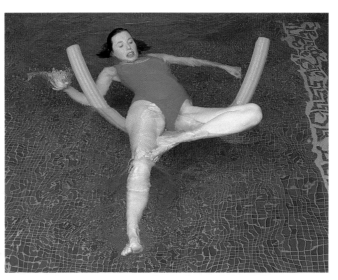

△ **1** Start by standing in the pool, holding the woggle behind your back. Lower it and lie down on your back with the woggle comfortably under you. Stretch your arms back over your head, palms together, and bend one leg, bringing your foot as high as you can go along the other leg without disturbing the alignment of your body.

△ **2** Alternatively, you can bend your leg first, holding on to the ends of the woggle and checking your alignment, before you stretch back and extend your arms above your head. Make sure your head is perfectly aligned in the pose.

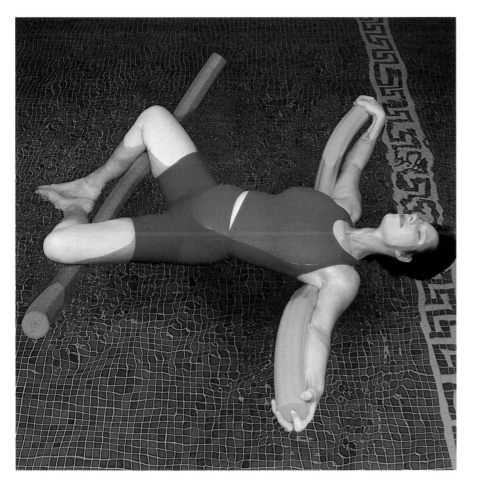

24 Floating butterfly pose

This is a restful, relaxing pose in which your pelvis is maximally open while your feet are joined, soles together. It is a good opportunity to enjoy the full benefits of classic yoga in the water during pregnancy, as this pose is reputed to be a panacea for women's health. Even if you float easily, having a woggle or board to support you will enable you to stretch and relax more in the pose. You can practise it throughout pregnancy, drawing a calm energy from it. Practise opening your legs wide and stretching them while you lie on your back in the water with your arms resting on a woggle in order to relax in the stretch, before you attempt the pose.

◁ **1** With a woggle supporting you behind your back and under your arms, stand facing a bar or a second woggle in front of you. Lower yourself in the water and place your bent legs over the bar or woggle, bringing the soles of your feet together and opening your knees wide. Stretch back, close to the surface of the water, resting your arms over the woggle on both sides. Let yourself completely relax in this supported floating pose and breathe deeply into your lower abdomen.

Dynamic stretches

This set of simple exercises is designed mainly for swimmers, or at least for those who are confident in water. They are aimed specifically at strengthening and lengthening the muscles that are used in swimming. The exercises are quite demanding and are intended for active, reasonably fit women who enjoy being in water. In these exercises, the resistance of the water against your body helps you deploy greater strength in the movement, yet with much greater freedom than in land-based yoga.

25 Full back stretch

In this rhythmic sequence, the whole body is stretched using simultaneous and alternate extensions and bends of the arms and legs. It is best done in a pool equipped with a bar along the side. You can do the symmetrical stretch holding on to a woggle but this does not give you as much resistance against which to stretch and bend your arms. You may launch yourself from the supported stretch into the floating one, either by pushing yourself off the pool wall or by letting go of the woggle and stretching back into a floating position. At first, while you are exploring your full stretch, you may find it helpful to keep your arm and leg slightly flexed for the asymmetrical stretch. Later, when this exercise is familiar to you, try to extend both arm and leg as fully as possible.

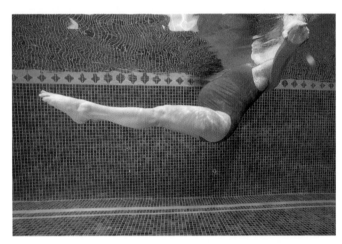

△ **1** Start with the supported, symmetrical stretch, even if you are a swimmer. Hold on to a woggle or the bar, breathe in and, as you breathe out, stretch out your arms and legs, extending your legs straight out together.

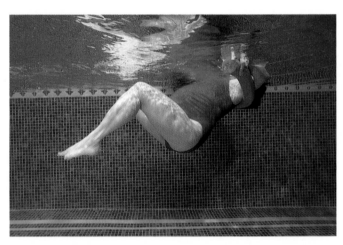

△ **2** Bend your legs and arms simultaneously on an in-breath and extend them on the next out-breath, getting into a steady energetic rhythm. This is quite tiring and you need to be careful not to exceed your optimal quota.

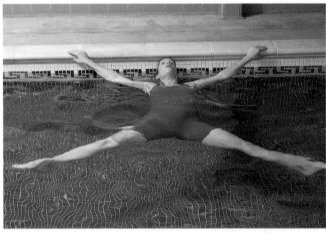

△ **3** Now open your legs as wide as possible and find a similar rhythmic movement in which you stretch further on each out-breath while keeping the whole sequence very relaxed. Some women find the version with legs open easier than the previous one, but both are equally demanding.

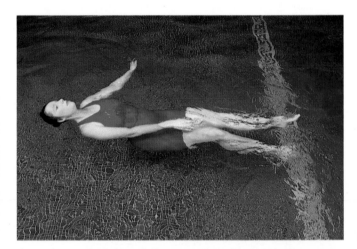

△ **4** For the asymmetrical stretch, float on your back with your arms along your body and your legs straight. You may use a woggle if you need support but try doing without one in this particular exercise as it can hamper your movement.

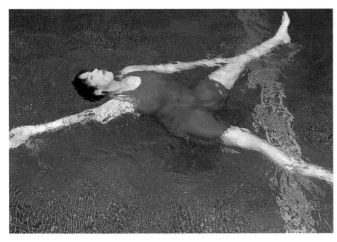

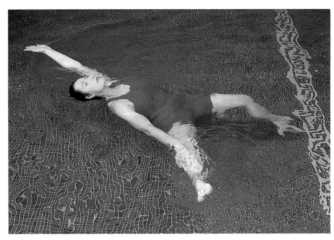

△ **5** As you inhale, open your left leg to the side and stretch your right arm behind you simultaneously. Stretch further as you breathe out.

△ **6** Bring your stretched arm and leg back to the centre as you breathe in again and immediately extend your other arm and leg in the same way as you breathe out. Continue to stretch alternating sides steadily with full cycles of your breath.

26 Back bend stretch

This sequence takes you from a back stretch to an open squat and back to the wall on your front. It can be as slow and relaxed or as fast and vigorous as you wish. Even in the vigorous mode, the mid-point of the sequence is totally relaxed as the body changes direction. This exercise tones the whole body and also improves your co-ordination. It is satisfying for the body and mind to experience a sense of loop in the sequence. If you are a confident swimmer, you may start your back stretch under water and return to the wall in a front stretch from your squatting position, pushing yourself from the pool floor to the pool wall. Skilled turns of freestyle swimmers against the wall can be seen as a closer, more rapid and advanced variation of this back bend, using the wall in the rotation phase rather than at the beginning of the sequence.

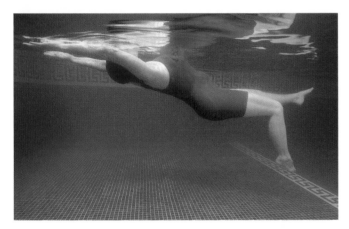

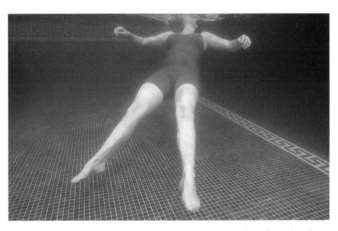

△ **1** Stand facing the pool wall and lower your body into the water by bending your legs. Inhale and push against the base of the wall with one leg, propelling yourself into the pool with a vigorous, yet relaxed, back stretch as you breathe out.

△ **2** Relax completely on the next flow of breath, letting your body lower itself again into the water.

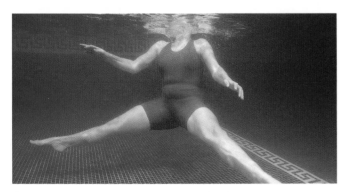

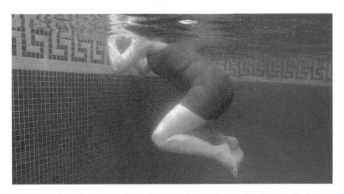

△ **3** Breathe in again and open your legs wide, with a vigorous movement.

△ **4** As you breathe out, bend your knees and rotate forward so that you find yourself close to a kneeling position in the water, facing the pool wall. You are now ready to start this exercise all over again.

Energetic stretches

Aqua yoga helps you to stretch vigorously and relax fully at the same time. Both stretching and relaxing are your best allies in preparing for the birth of your baby.

These energetic stretches invite you to combine both movement and complete relaxation. This corresponds not only to the essence of yoga but to the ways of many water animals, particularly water turtles and water mammals. Relaxed stretches both on the surface and under water will suit those who feel most at ease in water and enjoy going under the surface.

Simply do these stretches to your own rhythm. Pay close attention to the liberating and peaceful feelings of gliding relaxation and amphibian stretching which they will induce in you.

The vigorous start of the Water Turtle (27) helps launch you with momentum in to the submerged pose, while the Relaxed Roll Stretch (28) gives you a unique freedom of movement coupled with your own breathing rhythm. Make the most of these stretches: the water helps you enjoy the pleasurable feeling of your pregnant body in a way that would be impossible on dry land.

27 Water turtle

To start this sequence, in which the pose resembles that of a swimming water turtle, stand in the pool with your legs wide apart, your back straight and your arms along your body; breathe deeply.

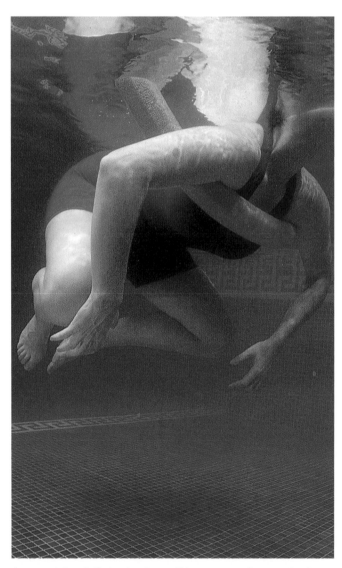

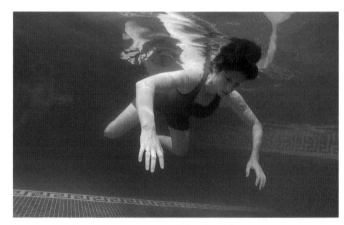

△ **2** Release your hands as you exhale, so that you find yourself in the water turtle pose. Sink slowly and land with your legs apart on the pool floor. Repeat the exercise a few times, paying attention to your breathing cycle.

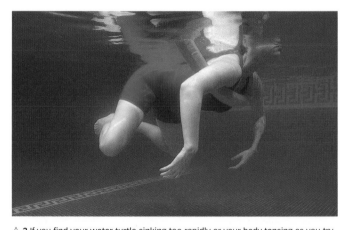

△ **3** If you find your water turtle sinking too rapidly or your body tensing as you try to reach your knees with your hands, try using a woggle under your arms. Instead of landing on the pool floor after taking your hands off your knees, you may choose to stretch forward along the surface of the water and touch your knees again from this position, opening and closing alternately as you swim like a turtle.

△ **1** On an in-breath, lift your bent legs as high as you can and rest your hands on your knees as you exhale. Shift your weight forward on the next in-breath.

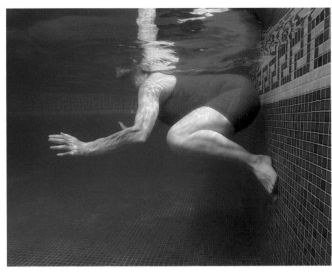

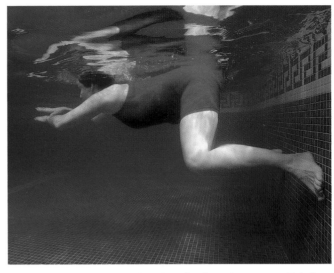

△ **4** If you are ready for a greater challenge, start from the wall, with your bent knees open, feet flat on the wall and your buttocks as close to the wall as possible. A vigorous breaststroke movement of your arms will keep you against the wall and make you breathe deeply in an intense open stretch.

△ **5** You can then push your legs from the wall and stretch your arms wide before relaxing and letting yourself go down towards the bottom of the pool like a water turtle. Stand up again when you are ready. This exercise is strenuous and repeating it twice is sufficient in one session.

28 Relaxed roll stretch

This swimming stretch will be very enjoyable for women who like moving in the water without using the particular skills of any given stroke. It is a free, flowing movement that can be done right up to the time of birth, making the most of water as a weight-free environment in which the constraints of late pregnancy can be forgotten for a while. Under water, the feeling of freedom is even greater. Although this exercise can also be done along the surface, it is difficult to roll sideways without putting your face in the water and those for whom this is not possible should not attempt it.

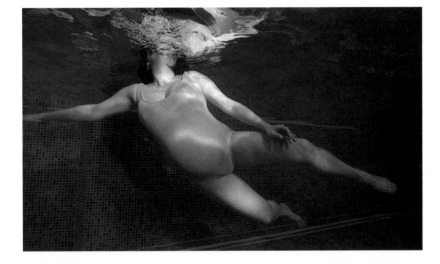

◁ **1** Stand with your back to the pool wall and knees bent. Lower your body and after taking a breath, push yourself off the wall with one foot, extending the arm on the same side. This is a relaxed stretch of your whole side.

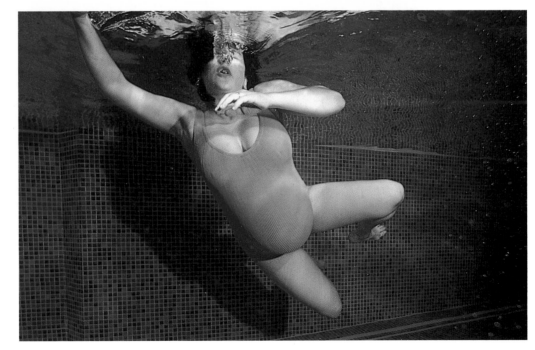

▷ **2** As you move away from the wall, blow out and, stretching your other arm back over your head in an overarm movement, roll on to your back, taking air again as you stretch. You can "roll-stretch" in this way a few times without getting tired if you keep your body relaxed in the movement.

Aqua yoga together

Aqua yoga, like yoga, is designed as an individual pursuit. However, it does not always have to be a solitary form of exercise. It can be done with friends both before and after birth. Here are a few examples of how friends and birth partners can help each other to stretch in aqua yoga, to their mutual benefit. Practising aqua yoga with a friend can considerably increase your confidence if you rely on the use of floats and woggles when you move away from the pool wall. It can also strengthen the non-verbal communication between birth partners that will be invaluable during labour.

If you have a toddler or small child who cannot quite swim yet, you can also involve him or her in part of your aqua yoga practice, holding on to you in the water.

Practising aqua yoga with your partner helps to strengthen the bonds between family members through this transformative time. Being in water facilitates the inevitably complex process of regression, adjustment and growth that the arrival of a new baby triggers in most families.

You can practise all the exercises in this book with a companion and find innovative ways of synchronizing and co-ordinating them. Here are just a few examples of what you can do.

29 Leg circles on the back

In this exercise, friends take turn to stretch each other. The pregnant woman, supported by one or two floats under each arm, is stretched on her back by either a standing or a swimming helper, who moves her legs in wide circles. If you are not totally water-confident, it is best to start with the standing version. You need more space to do the swimming version, as both you and your helper move in the water with your bodies extended.

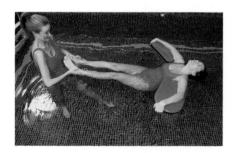

△ **1** Get into a stable supported position on your back in the water before your helper takes hold of your feet. This is a passive exercise where the movement is done for you. Let go and enjoy it completely, focusing on breathing as deeply as possible.

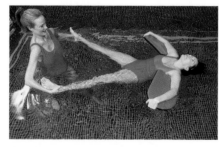

△ **2** Your helper starts circling your legs as wide as possible, bending the knees and stretching the legs in a wide breaststroke movement.

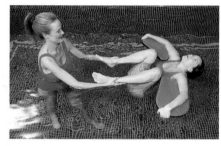

△ **3** Guide your helper if necessary to find the steady, slow, smooth rhythm that suits you best. If the helper also breathes fully at the same time, this can be an equally good exercise of the arms and shoulders.

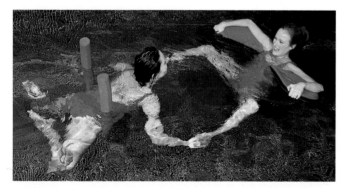

△ **4** If your helper is also pregnant she can use a woggle to gain as much from the swimming version of the exercise as you. Your starting position is as before, but the helper is more immersed, with the woggle in place, standing with bent knees so that her arm movement is on the surface of the water in line with your leg circling. Once a suitable rhythm has been found, the helper can take off, synchronizing a slow breaststroke with the outward stretching of your legs.

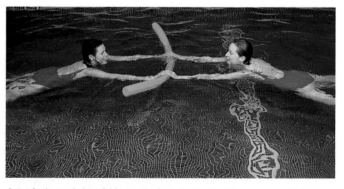

△ **5** A further variation of this exercise is a joint breaststroke leg movement in which the two of you hold a woggle on either side, so that you exert a resistance against each other as you stretch together.

30 Joint floating stretch

Stretching side by side with a friend can be a very enjoyable shared experience. Joint floating stretches and relaxation can deepen non-verbal communication between friends and promote friendship, enhancing the individual experience of each woman in a non-competitive, relaxing way. Drifting along may bring friends close together and apart again.

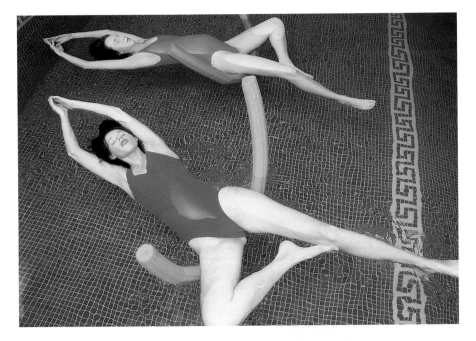

◁ **1** Use a woggle each to support the base of your thighs, protect your lower back in a full stretch and ease your floating. Extend your arms back over your head on an inhalation. As you exhale, bend one knee and bring your foot against the inner side of the other leg, which remains extended on the surface of the water. Breathe fully as you continue stretching and relaxing at the same time, enjoying both the stillness and the extension of your body, which is pure yoga. Change legs and repeat on the other side. To end this exercise, bring your arms to the side and along your body and lower your pelvis in the water into a half-sitting position so that you can remove your woggle easily and stand up. You can also extend your bent leg and get into a floating relaxation directly from this stretch.

31 Involve your toddler

A woggle under your arms, at the front or at the back, will give you enough extra buoyancy not to mind having a toddler hanging on to you while you are doing aqua yoga exercises. A couple of stretches are shown here to inspire you but, with the exception of the stretch-bends and swings, most of the exercises in this book can be done with a toddler in tow. It helps if he or she is water-confident and does not mind going under occasionally.

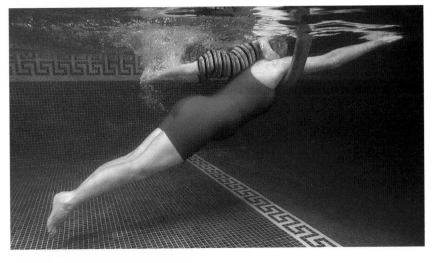

▷ **1** Try a full stretch, propelling your body forward with either a frog kick or by pushing your feet off the floor.

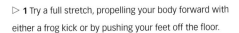

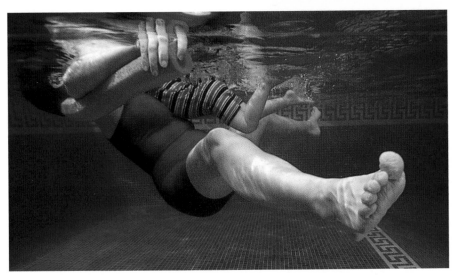

◁ **2** Your toddler can sit on you while you are lying back, supporting yourself on one or two woggles. This gives you the freedom to stretch your legs wide and then bend them, which opens your pelvis. Circle your legs if you can: you might not be able to extend your body as much as if you were on your own but you may share a lot of fun with your child.

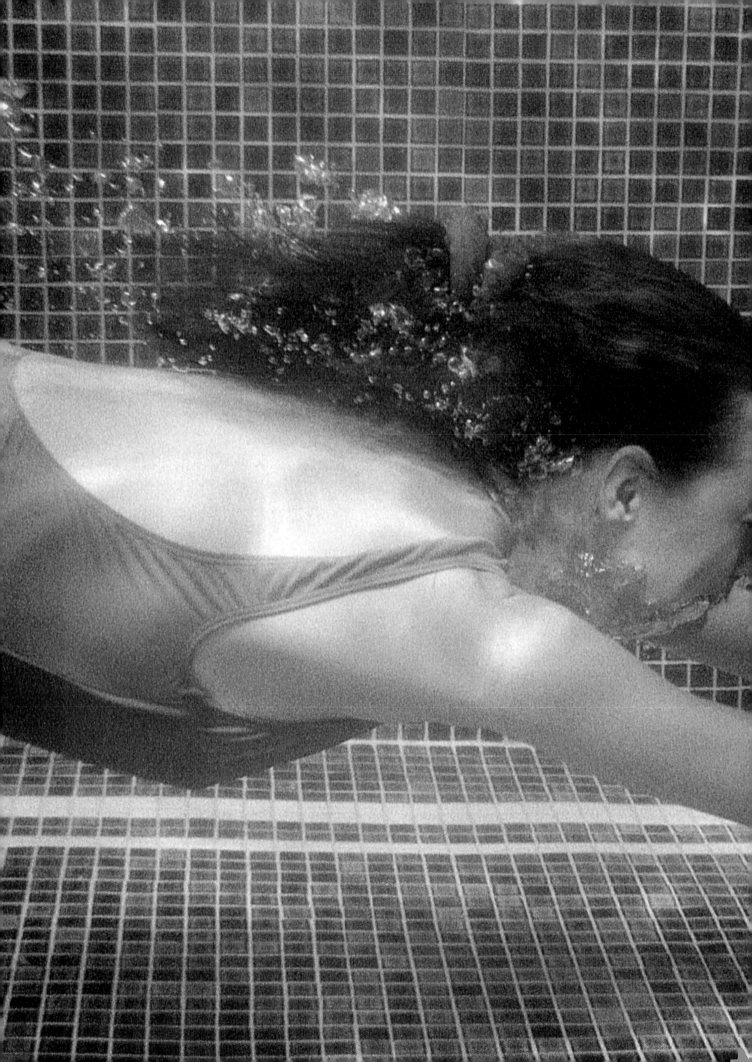

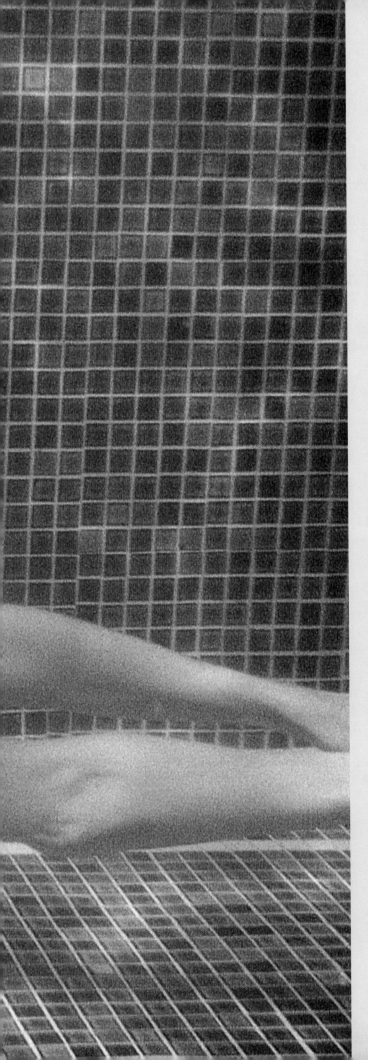

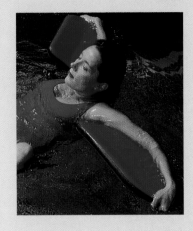

antenatal
swimming

Throughout pregnancy, aqua yoga swimming

opens the pelvis and stretches the whole body,

elongating the spine and expanding the breathing

capacity. The focus is not on speed but on

maximum relaxed stretching, full use of your

breathing and a symmetrical use of joints and

muscles. You are actually encouraged to swim

extremely slowly, yet with an efficient technique

that aims at generating a very smooth rhythm and

movement. All sequences are designed for all stages

of pregnancy unless stated otherwise.

Adapted breaststroke swimming

Swimming is excellent for breath control, and adapted breaststroke in pregnancy encourages you to breathe using your diaphragm more effectively. Emphasis is placed on the exhalation phase during the forward thrust, ideally with your face in the water. This will ensure a smoother rhythm and eliminate any forced or jerky movements of the legs. The minimum amount of energy is used, while greater precision and a smoother movement is achieved.

If you wish to swim breaststroke without support, it is best to do so with your face in the water. Keeping your head above the water makes it impossible for you to open the pelvis in the way that makes breaststroke valuable during pregnancy. It also places strain on the muscles at the base of the neck.

If you learnt to swim breaststroke a long time ago and never explored how to breathe, now is your opportunity to do so, at the same time acquiring a more precise and efficient technique with a fully aligned spine.

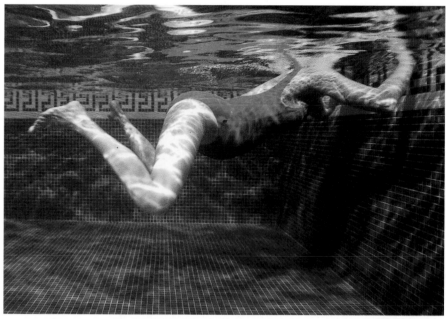

△You can check the breaststroke leg action at the bar first. If you learnt how to swim this stroke as a child, the triple action of opening your knees, stretching your legs open and bringing your knees under your body again will return to you easily. Feel the effect of this movement on your pregnant body and explore the rhythm that suits you best as you focus on your breathing at the same time.

32 Water-boatwoman

This exercise resembles the action of the insects called water-boatmen on the surface of ponds. The resistance of the water to your whole body is decreased to an absolute minimum. Ideally you should hardly move forward at all, while you feel more and more spread out on the surface of the water in a floating movement in which your hips open wider and wider.

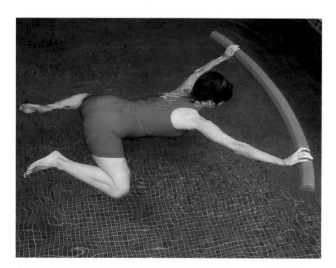

△ **1** Propel your body with a very wide breaststroke leg movement while your upper body remains relaxed, supported on floats. Your pelvis is open, your buttocks raised and your supported arms open. Raise your knees as much as possible, to achieve a very wide circle close to the surface. This can also be done with floats under each arm for support.

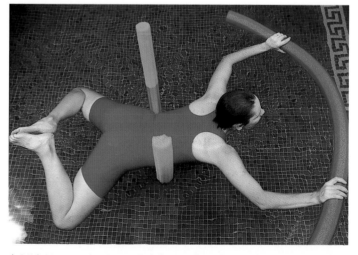

△ **2** Using two woggles as supports helps you align your upper body along the surface of the water while you focus on the leg movement. From a nearly static "water-boatwoman", you can extend your legs more, propelling yourself in the water with a strong yet flowing movement, avoiding the uneven action of the legs that can make breaststroke swimming uncomfortable.

33 Aqua yoga breaststroke

Once you have achieved a smooth circling of the legs with your arms supported in the "water-boatwoman" exercise, you are ready to synchronize the arm and leg movements of breaststroke. Most of the propulsion comes from the legs but the emphasis is on the lateral stretch rather than on a forward motion. The arm movement opens the chest in a way that helps to expand your breathing and uplift your spirit.If you have been swimming competition-style breaststroke before pregnancy, the challenge now is to lengthen your whole spine along the surface of the water rather than raising your upper back out of the water as you inhale and propel yourself. Start swimming very slowly and consider it as a different stroke – one for stretch rather than speed. It is an extended exhalation in the stretch that will enable you to discover the "yoga of swimming": minimum expenditure of energy with a fulfilling rhythm in an increasingly efficient stroke.

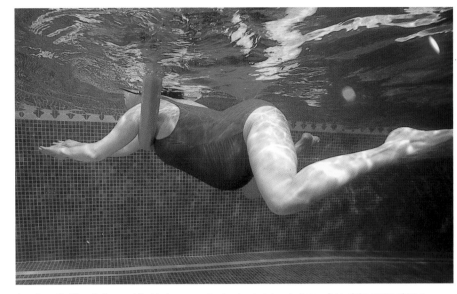

△ **1** If you find it a challenge at first to keep your back extended close to the surface of the water, place a woggle under your arms for additional support. With your shoulders and neck relaxed, focus on synchronizing your breathing with a broad, regular movement of your arms and legs. Allow a long, gliding stretch before bringing your arms back and bending your knees open to propel yourself forward again, extending both your breathing cycle and your movement at the same time.

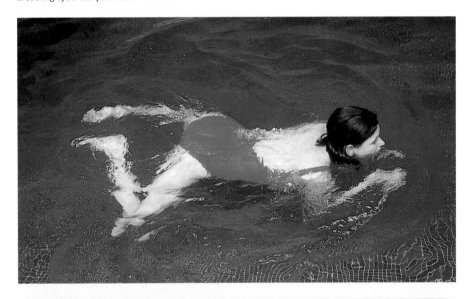

▷ **2** Stand with your back against the pool wall. Bend your knees and extend your arms forward, inhaling as you propel yourself away from the pool wall. Take two long strokes with your mouth or your whole face in the water, inhaling on the second stroke. Aim to stretch the front of your body as much as possible, extending the gliding forward thrust of each stroke as far as you can.

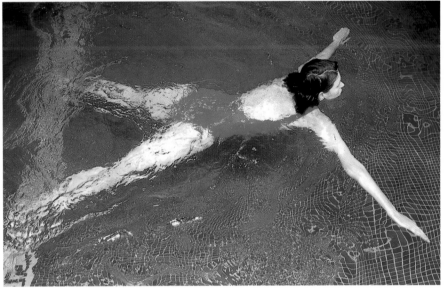

▷ **3** Raise your head and inhale again as you bring your arms back at the end of the second stroke. The most effective head position is with the waterline about mid-forehead, raising the head just enough to inhale – through the nose or more often through the mouth – and then exhale under the surface. Aim at a smooth forward movement in which there is virtually no gap between your arm stretch and your arm pull, your in-breath and your out-breath.

Adapted backstroke

This stroke is ideal if you feel you stretch best on your back but can no longer do so in late pregnancy. It is also a good stroke if you do not like putting your face in the water and can be "swum" by non-swimmers if supported with woggles or floats. Whether you are a swimmer or not, supported aqua yoga backstroke is an essential aquacise during pregnancy, opening the pelvis and toning the muscles that support the growing baby and that are used in childbirth.

As in breaststroke, the aim during pregnancy is to improve relaxation in the swimming movement so that the energy expended is reduced and a greater stretch is achieved in a steady, slow rhythm of deep breathing. This in turn leads to further relaxed stretching and greater efficiency of movement and breathing combined.

Whether you are using your arms or not, when swimming on your back, check that you remain as streamlined as possible. Let the water support your head and back together, getting into your stroke from the pleasure of floating.

Even if you are not a backstroke swimmer, you can still enjoy unsupported swimming on your back. Try using your arms and hands to keep your upper body on the surface of the water with a sculling action under water, while your legs and feet propel you just as when you were supported by the floats. If you find yourself sitting and sinking rather than taking off on your back, don't get discouraged. Part of becoming a mother is giving up being an overachiever; take it easy and welcome successes and setbacks as an ongoing process.

Symmetrical backstroke

Once you can move freely in the water on your back, you can practise an open, symmetrical backstroke known in swimming circles as the "English backstroke". This is an excellent stroke for pregnancy although it has fallen into disuse due to the greater effectiveness of the back crawl.

In this stroke, propulsion through the water is created through the movement of your arms and hands and your legs and feet in a symmetrical, synchronized stretching and circling. Inhale as you open your arms as widely as possible behind you and at the same time open your knees as in the supported backstroke. Exhale as you bring your arms back to the centre. Make this a wide, flowing movement.

Although it is energetic, there is no need for huge splashes. Try to keep your body close to the water surface. At first, there is a tendency to sink the pelvis and heave your arms back instead of lifting them in a smooth movement. Then you may feel that the rhythm of the stroke propels you without the need to raise your body up and backwards in the overarm action.

Back crawl

If you can, swim backstroke with an alternating arm pull. This is known as back crawl. Keep a good balance and fluent action to maintain the balance of your body through the stroke. This will help you to elongate your back muscles in your early to mid pregnancy. It is important to position your head so that your ears are in the water and your neck feels relaxed. Your arms should move freely over the side and then along your body with a relaxed stretch. Keep your leg-kicks light and just below the surface of the water. In late pregnancy, it may become more difficult to preserve your balance as your body rolls with the alternate arm action. In that case, focus on the Backstroke Leg Circles (35) until you can resume the back crawl again after the birth.

34 Back rowing

This exercise uses the resistance of the water to tone arm and shoulder muscles as well as the muscles that support the breasts. The blood flow to and from these muscles is increased and the lymph nodes in the armpits, which may be very sensitive during pregnancy, are better drained.

Back rowing also improves your capacity to relax and it is a good exercise to practice if you have only a short time in the pool and are feeling agitated and stressed when you arrive.

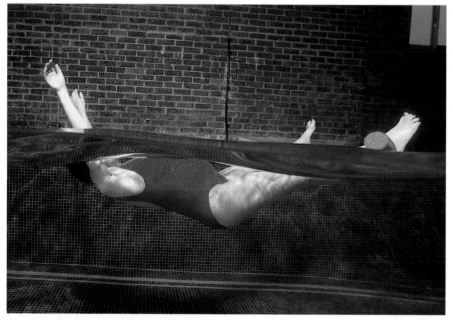

△ 1 With your feet under the bar or resting on a woggle, lift your arms back over your head, opening them wide in a circling movement.

35 Backstroke leg circles

The propulsion created by your legs and feet pushes the water behind you in this stroke, with a vigorous yet harmonious circling movement of the hips and knees while the upper body is supported on floats or woggles. At first, give priority to your leg movement and do not worry if you find yourself half sitting in the water. As you become familiar with the exercise, stretch your back as much as you can along the surface of the water.

▷ **1** Your pelvis should be open, your knees turned out (not tucked up), your chest open and your head relaxed, with your chin tucked in. Breathe out as you pull your legs in towards your body and inhale as you open them out again.

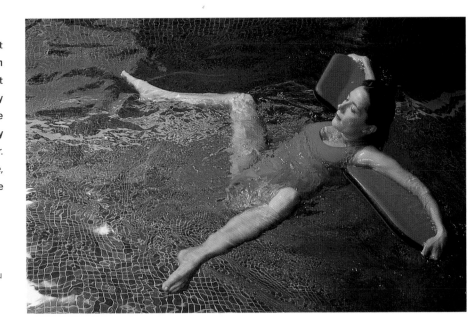

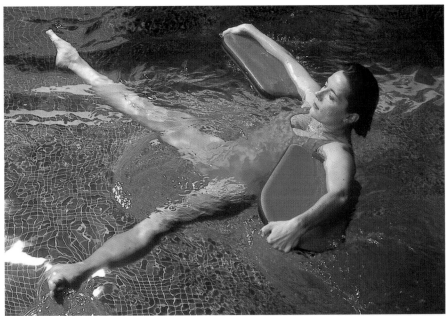

◁ **2** To relax and stretch your legs at the same time after practising your backstroke leg circles, alternately extend one leg while bending the other, using a relaxed kicking movement just under the surface of the water with your ankles relaxed.

▷ **3** If you have practised backstroke leg circles or back rowing as a main component of your session, always relax in a floating position afterwards. Use woggles or floats to align your whole body on the surface of the water, with your legs stretched open. Breathe deeply into your abdomen, allowing your heartbeat to return to normal, then enjoy a relaxing floating stretch for a few seconds.

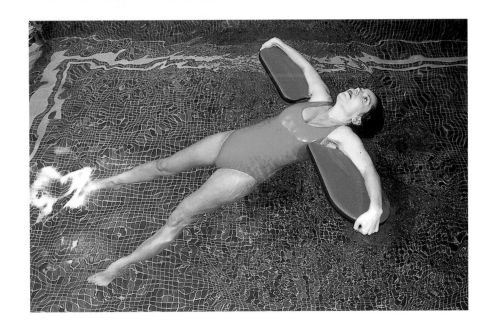

Freestyle swimming

Crawl is suitable during pregnancy if you are a good swimmer and this is your stroke of choice. Also, if you are expecting your third baby (or more) and you still feel stretched from your previous pregnancy, the crawl can tone your abdominal muscles before you begin stretching again, particularly in early and mid-pregnancy. How well these strokes serve you during your pregnancy depends on how much you can incorporate your breathing into the stroke cycle. In late pregnancy, when you are preparing to give birth, it is best to give priority to breaststroke and basic backstroke in your practice. The butterfly stroke is only appropriate in early to mid pregnancy if it is your favourite stroke. The dolphin dives are suitable throughout pregnancy.

36 Front and back crawl

Keeping a good balance is important in the crawl when you are pregnant. Controlling your breathing pattern and improving your rhythm helps you adjust your balance as you grow larger each month so that you do not develop lateral body movements or excessive rolling from side to side. Swim with a continuous, flowing action, keeping your head and neck relaxed as you turn to breathe.

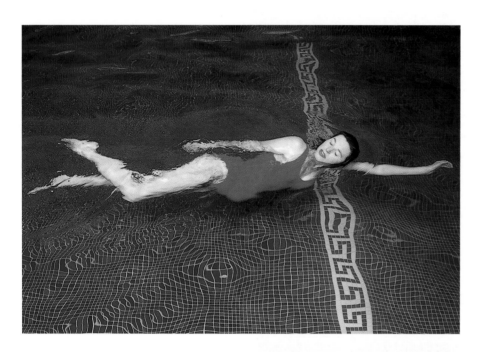

◁ **1** Stretch as much as possible on the surface of the water, steamlining your body and keeping your legs and ankles relaxed as you kick. Avoid making a splash with your feet; your movement is more efficient if they remain just below the surface, without actually breaking it, at all times.

▷ **2** In the alternate overarm action of the back crawl, a relaxed stretching of each arm in turn along the ear is very pleasant in mid to late pregnancy as it extends the whole body better and more safely than could be achieved lying down. Keep the flutter kick relaxed, knees straight but not tense, with the movement coming mainly from the ankles. Ideally your chin would be tucked in but in this relaxed version, just make sure that your head is not extending back. If you are able to see the edge of the pool, or, even better, your feet, you will be streamlined enough to enjoy breathing freely in the stroke, experiencing a balanced, relaxed, pleasurable stretch in your own rhythm.

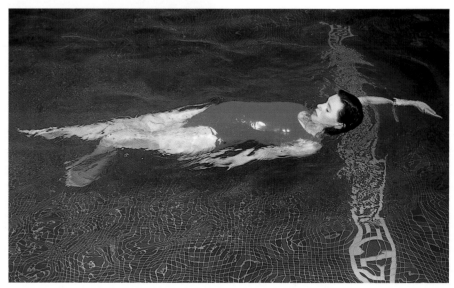

37 Dolphin dives

The butterfly stroke is the basis for Dolphin Dives and requires the most physical strength of all swimming strokes. It carries the risk of exaggerating the lumbar curve of your spine – even more so as your uterus grows. If you are a keen swimmer and it is your favourite stroke, you can continue to enjoy swimming it in early to mid pregnancy, but do not attempt it otherwise. Dolphin Dives are different. They are a safe, adapted version of the butterfly and protect your lower back. The combined action of breath and movement make it a streamlined stretch, effective and easy to practise in a pool where the water is shoulder deep. Dolphin Dives single out and accentuate the diving and emerging actions in the butterfly stroke but do not need the strength or skill to propel the body through the leg and back movement. You can also vary the depths of your dives, from just below the surface to the bottom of the pool. With little expenditure of energy, you can exercise all the muscles of your back in just a few minutes of dives.

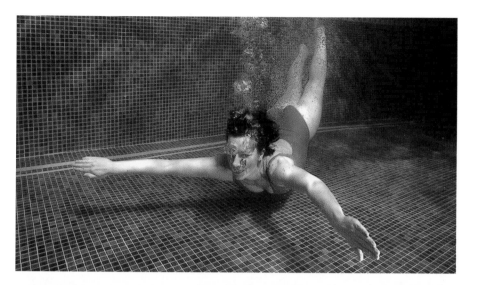

◁ **1** Standing in the water, extend your arms in front of you and, rounding your back, flex your legs and jump to dive. Either trail your extended legs as you move down and up or use the flipper leg motion of the butterfly stroke to propel you.

▽ **2** Take your arms back slowly to your sides as your body follows the trajectory of the dive down then back up to the surface. In a shallow pool you can stretch along the pool floor before coming back up, all in one long breath. As you come up, open your arms out to the side, then extend them in front of you and take another dive.

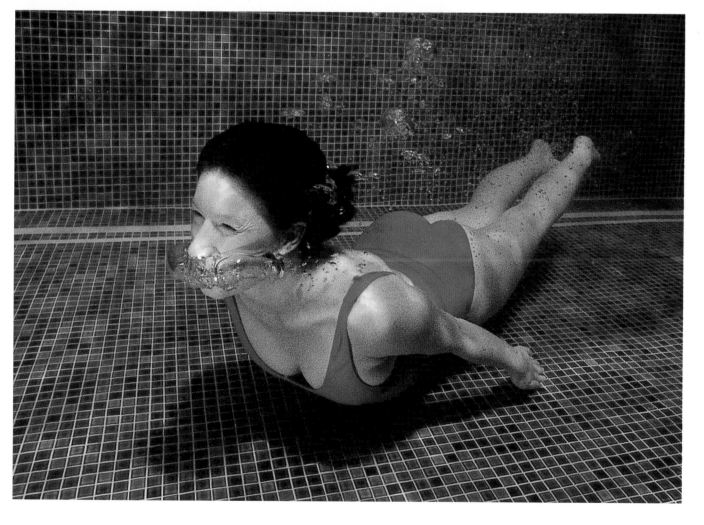

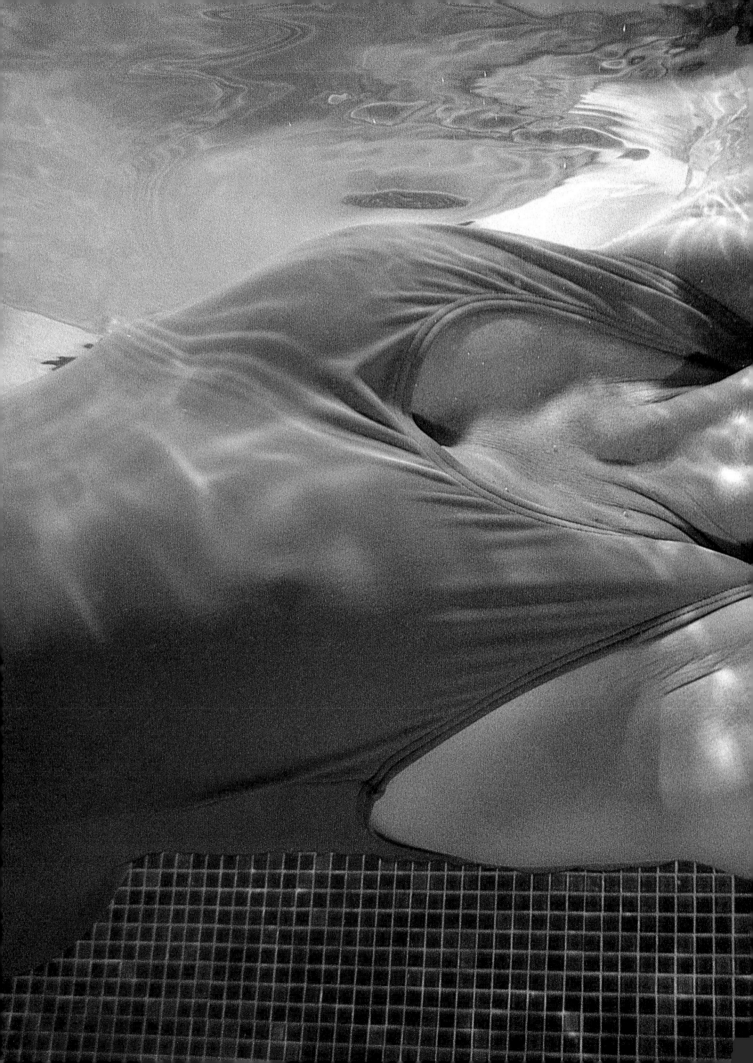

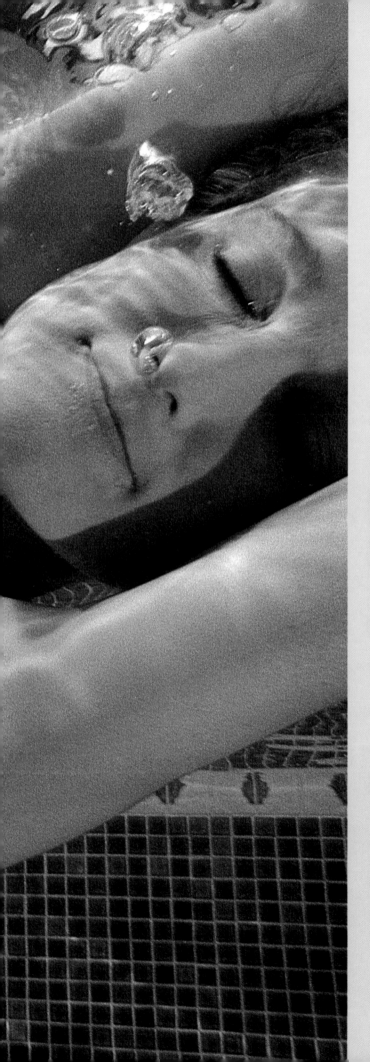

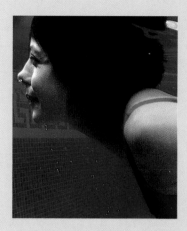

antenatal
breathing &
relaxation

The effortless extension of the body in water

allows an expansion of the breath that can

otherwise only be achieved through a longer

period of practice, either of lane swimming or of

yoga. Full abdominal breathing in pregnancy also

benefits the unborn child. If water is to be used

in labour, as a safe and effective method of

relieving pain, it is best to start expanding the

breath as early as possible.

The breath of life

When you practise this diving exercise, your body comes to terms with unspoken fears such as running out of oxygen, drowning, failing or exhaustion. These are the same fears that you are likely to experience in labour during long contractions. Use the aqua breathing to find a way to relax while in the grip of these deep-seated fears. It can transform the frightening experience and is an extremely useful aid during labour.

Gaining further and easier forward movement in your long dive is not just an inspiration for your labour, but is an actual practice for your body, a physical training to help you to deal with these sensations in a postive way. Bodies learn fast and yours will reward you for this practice.

All women who have done this exercise in pregnancy use it in a positive way during their labour. For many, it has transformed their experience of giving birth.

38 Breathing dives with relaxation

Breathing dives can be done on the surface or underwater, or using a combination of both. Underwater dives are more effective, not only because the body is freer in the water but also because the mind enters another world. In a few seconds, a different state of consciousness can be reached. It can also be left behind easily as the body re-emerges into the activity of the pool. Start relaxing as soon as you emerge.

It helps to do this exercise with a partner, who can give you a little push when you are learning to release more movement from your relaxed stretch, or just cheer as you go further and further each time and finally cross the pool. Once you have found the way to continue your initial movement effortlessly, relax as you extend your exhalation to the maximum of your breathing capacity. The distances between your starting and finishing points will surprise you.

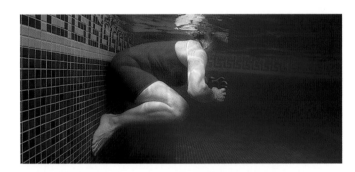

◁ **1** Start in a semi-squat position against the pool wall, ready to propel yourself forward by pushing your feet against the wall.

▽ **2** Take a breath and, with a strong push from your feet at the base of the wall, stretch as much as you can in a long dive.

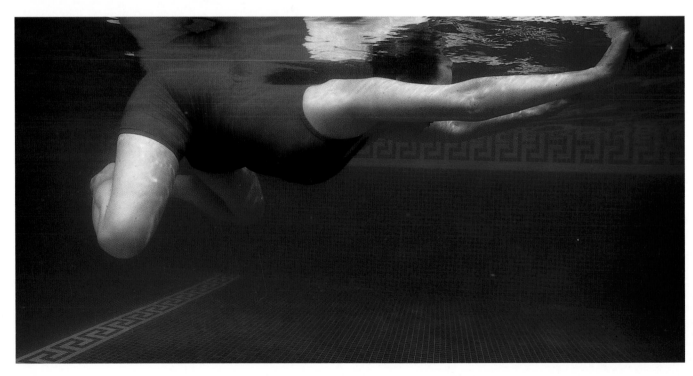

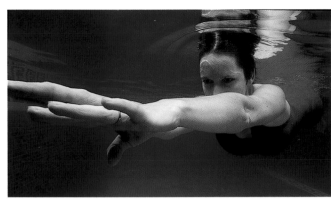

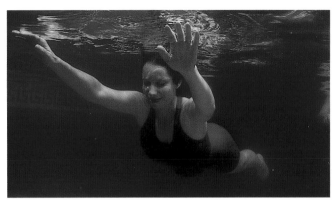

△ **3** Streamline your body as much as possible to diminish the resistance of the water as you push forward, relying on kinetic energy to take you as far as possible. The more you relax in a streamlined stretch, the less additional resistance is created and the further you reach.

△ **4** The challenge is to learn to relax more as you feel the urge to raise your head and breathe. Relax your whole body. You may find yourself sinking, or going to one side, even going into a full circle. Let it happen. Register your feelings. Do not struggle, but when you cannot let go any longer, surface and breathe deeply.

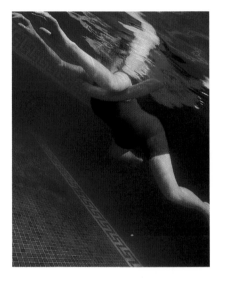

◁ **5** If you find that your legs start sinking as soon as your head and shoulders emerge from the water, place a woggle under your arms. Often it gives you just the support you need to avoid tensing up and to fully enjoy deepening your breathing as you stretch.

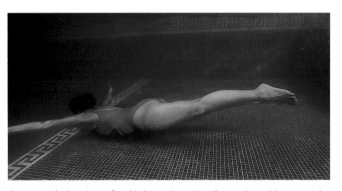

△ **6** As you feel more comfortable in your breathing dives and are able to extend them and relax in them, you can stretch close to the bottom of the pool in a deeper dive. In doing so you become even more at one with the waterworld of fairy tales and myths for a moment, with all its creative potential. Many pregnant women experience this as an environment in which they can feel freer.

▷ **7** Some women feel more comfortable taking dives with their arms running along their bodies rather than outstretched. If you have a tendency to high blood pressure and try to avoid raising your arms on dry land, this version may also be more appropriate for you. It is important to keep your neck and head relaxed in the forward movement.

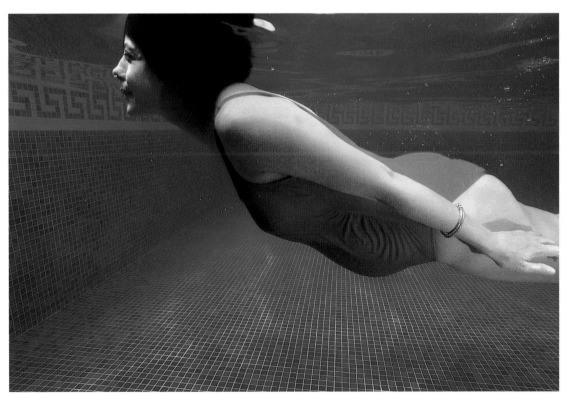

Floating relaxation

If you have already tried the adapted strokes described earlier in this book, you will have found that when you use the breath fully in swimming and make your movement as economical as possible, you become more relaxed. Within a very short time, you have forgotten the concerns, worries, and even anxieties, that are inevitable as you go through pregnancy. By the time you get out of the pool, many preoccupations will have been reduced to a manageable scale. Anxiety is the greatest unacknowledged discomfort that prevents most women from enjoying their pregnancies fully. Relaxing in water is both the best prevention and cure and can be achieved easily.

The benefits of relaxation

Floating is an extremely powerful form of relaxation. Relaxation encompasses your body, mind and emotions. Its physiological effects include a lower heart rate and blood pressure, a lower respiratory rate, lower blood cortizone level and the production of theta and alpha brainwaves. As these brainwave patterns are produced, emotions – from yesterday or many years back – can be triggered by sensory or mental stimuli to surface in the psyche.

The floating relaxation recommended here is gentle and safe. During pregnancy it can nevertheless result in the release of pent-up emotions, either positive or negative, and have a cathartic effect. For this reason it is important to follow the instructions carefully and, particularly in the last few weeks

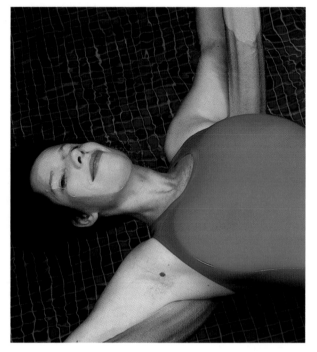

◁ In the same way that relaxation integrates and draws together the benefits of stretching in land-based yoga postures, floating relaxation is essential to the practice of aqua yoga. Floating relaxation can be practised on your own or with a partner. Except for very experienced swimmers who can relax in water without support, it is best done with floats, woggles or human hands to help you float effortlessly.

of pregnancy, it is preferable to relax in water with someone else, ideally the person who will be with you during labour.

Floating relaxation is an effective way to learn to relax quickly during pregnancy if you have not practised relaxation before. The more you practise, the more effective it becomes, as the relaxed body sends signals to the brain which in turn sends more signals of relaxation to the body. If you are familiar with yoga, you will find that floating will deepen your experience and also enrich your yogic relaxation. In the water, it is easy to access quite rapidly levels of relaxation that are normally reached through the apprenticeship of "withdrawing the senses"

(pratyahara) in yoga practice. The earlier in pregnancy you start the floating relaxation, the more benefit you will derive from it during labour and later on, as you gain the ability to centre yourself instantly, either to draw upon your inner resources or to let yourself go into deep sleep after being woken up by your baby. Relaxation in water also enhances the rise in endorphin levels during the latter part of pregnancy, producing a sense of wellbeing and suppressing undue anxiety as the due date draws near.

Supported relaxation

Although greater buoyancy is released as the supported woman relaxes more deeply, the action of supporting requires some strength. Particularly when two pregnant women are helping each other, you should take time to ensure that supporting is as beneficial as being supported. It is a good idea to take turns to experience the two roles and to learn to relax as a supporter as well. Ideally, both are complementary in the experience. Allow approximately 5 minutes of relaxation at first, 5–10 minutes when you have gained experience.

Theta brainwaves

Theta brainwaves are produced in deep relaxation or when we are absorbed in daydreaming. Brainwave patterns have been detected in foetuses as early as the fifth week. By the time the baby is born, brainwaves are mostly theta or delta (daydreaming or sleeping) until they change gradually into the normal beta rhythm that indicates a greater focus on the external world. Floating relaxation may induce theta waves in a pregnant woman's brain and in turn allow her baby to produce more theta waves. Its regular practice may continue to have a calming effect on the baby in the first year.

39 Relaxation with a partner

In early and mid-pregnancy, it is ideal to practise floating relaxation with a pregnant friend as regularly as possible, ideally once a week. In late pregnancy, your labour partner, whether the father-to-be or someone else, can also begin to support you in the water as a way to deepen the unspoken communication that may prove to be most valuable to you at the time of birth. If two pregnant women are partners in the floating relaxation, they may find that their respective babies are involved too, and sometimes show it by their simultaneous movement in the womb.

It is best to swim a little after floating relaxation before getting out of the pool. If you are not a swimmer, do a few drops at the bar or practise your favourite swings or rolls. In late pregnancy be very careful if you have to drive away from the pool. Take time to allow your body to come back to active mode. After having a shower, practise Alternate Nostril Breathing (1) for a couple of minutes. Ideally, sit down and have a healthy drink and snack before leaving.

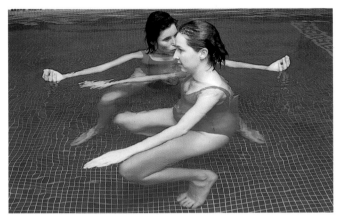

△ **1** The position of the supporting person is very important. As the supporter, you should stand with your knees slightly bent so that your back is straight and your body is relaxed with a solid base. You will be supporting the relaxing woman with your arms, yet the source of the support will be your lower back. Once the supporter is in a strong open standing position, the relaxing woman lowers her body so that she is nearly sitting in the water. If the supporter is right-handed, the relaxing woman should sit sideways with her legs to the right, as the strong hand of the supporter will be under her lower back taking most of the weight. If the supporter is left-handed, the pregnant woman faces the left of the supporter.

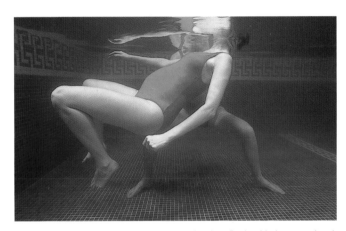

△ **2** Adjust your positions so that support can be given firmly with the strong hand under the lower back and the other hand at the base of the neck. With hands in place, the supporter assists the relaxing woman to swivel into a lying position as effortlessly as possible. There is always a point that feels right and most comfortable for both of you, at which stage the relaxation can begin.

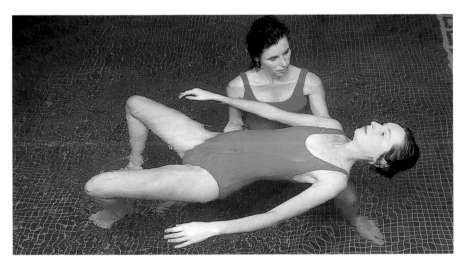

△ **3** If you are the supporter, check that the pregnant woman's body is level just below the surface, with her legs hanging loosely or floating. At first, rocking her body from side to side can help her start relaxing, while her eyes are still open. Encourage her to exhale consciously several times to achieve a state of deep relaxation. She can then close her eyes. Check that her ears are in the water so that only her face is emerging. From then on, you as the supporter will relax too, yet keeping a watch on the pregnant woman. If she shows discomfort and stirs, lower your hand under her back immediately to bring her back to a standing position; if you experience discomfort or feel tense in holding her, do the same, as any tension will inevitably be communicated to her.

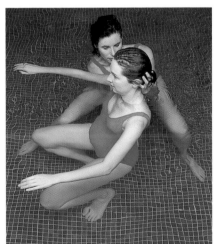

△ **4** The floating woman will need 2–5 minutes to get her body back in focus, sometimes longer in late pregnancy. The supporting partner can keep the hand under the base of the neck in place to help her do this at her own pace.

Just you and your baby

Self-supporting floating relaxation can be a time of exceptional intimacy with your baby, in which you experience each other without any external stimuli and with less of the usual train of thought that keeps the mind engaged in all the activities of the day. It allows you to reach a deeper state in which superficial worries and anxieties have no hold. The sheer magic of the little being growing inside becomes more congenial and can be experienced in the present moment just as it is. This experience may facilitate bonding at the time of birth.

Drifting

As you relax you may find yourself drifting in the pool, sometimes even a considerable distance from your point of departure. If you are relaxed, you will not hurt yourself if you hit the pool wall while you drift, although it may bring you out of your relaxation in an untimely way.

With practice you will learn to control your drifting by relaxing more deeply: the deeper your relaxation, the less you will move. This is another reason why it is better to relax with a friend at first if you can, as he or she can gently look after you while you relax. There is no timekeeping when you are on your own and some women have spent half an hour floating while feeling that barely a couple of minutes had passed.

Relaxation and release

If you connect with past traumas or painful memories while you are practising floating relaxation on your own, try to talk about your experience with someone you trust. This will help you decide whether you need to seek further help to address the experience in a positive way.

In Ayurveda, the ancient medical system associated with yoga, pregnancy is seen as the greatest purifying process the human physiology can experience. Deep relaxation during pregnancy allows the possible resolution of difficult past experiences,

Be safe!

Self-supporting floating relaxation should be practised with a lifeguard on site, or at least with someone watching at all times.

particularly miscarriages and pregnancy terminations, which can compromise the full enjoyment of pregnancy for many women. In the intimately comforting environment that water provides, floating relaxation is a gentle yet very effective way of letting go of past experiences and simply being with this growing baby or babies in the fullness of the present moment.

Using supports

If you do not have access to woggles, use one or two floats under each arm. It is possible that your legs will sink down as you relax. You may use another float under your feet, though it can be difficult to hold it in place, or let your legs dangle down in the water.

You will find relaxing easier and more comfortable with woggles than with floats and there are various ways you can use them. Experiment to find the way that suits you best and allows you to close your eyes and relax deeply. If you are not water-confident and need more support to feel safe while floating, a second woggle can be added to one placed under the arms.

40 With one woggle under the knees, holding on

Many women like the sense of control that this position gives them as they can let go and relax in their own time. If they are interrupted they have only to lower their bodies in to the water keeping the ends of the woggle in their hands. Others find holding the woggle a constraint that limits the depth of their relaxation in the water.

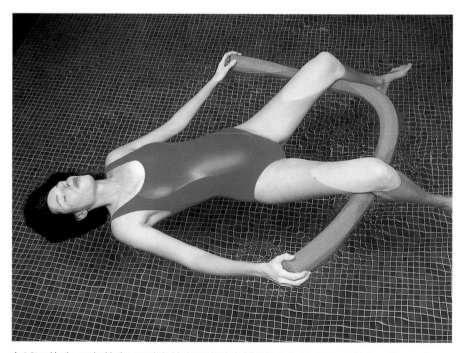

△ **1** Stand in the pool with the woggle behind your back, holding its ends. Lower yourself into a sitting position and bring the woggle under your thighs. Stretch back so that your whole trunk can be on the surface of the water. Open your knees slightly and find a comfortable position in which you can be most relaxed, extending your legs only to the point where your arms are not stretching to hold the woggle. Once you have found this balance, let go and close your eyes, keeping your ears in the water and your face above the surface.

41 With two woggles, holding on

You can use an additional woggle under your shoulders and arms as you hold your main supporting woggle under your bent knees. This gives you complete support, yet still some control as you continue to hold the woggles at their junction. It also gives extra support to your neck and creates a comforting ring in which you can be less easily disturbed in a public pool.

▷ **1** Have the second woggle under your arms so that when you lower your body to pass the first woggle under your knees, it stays in place for you to spread your arms on and then join the two woggles together.

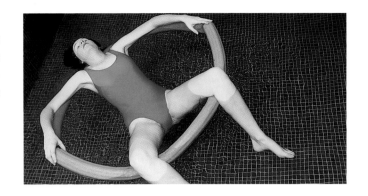

42 With one woggle under the knees, letting go

If possible allow space around you when you start relaxing or be prepared for the risk of being interrupted. Remember that it is not advisable to practise floating relaxation on your own in a pool without a lifeguard on duty.

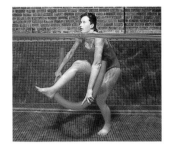

△ **1** Stand in the water holding a woggle in front of you and lower it in the water. Bend one leg and lift it so that you can pass the woggle under it.

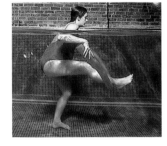

△ **2** Lift your leg higher as you lower your body in the water, which makes it easy to bring your other leg on top of the woggle.

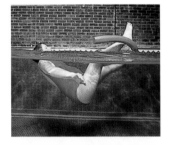

◁ **3** Now you can release your hands and lean back, with the woggle in place under your ankles, looking at your feet on the surface of the pool. At this stage, you may be in a reclined position, half sitting in the water.

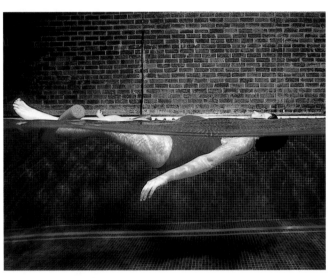

△ **4** Take a breath and as you exhale, stretch back and let go more so that just your face is out of the water. You can now start relaxing deeply, closing your eyes. Let your ears submerge and, if comfortable, lower your head so that just your nose and eyes are above the surface. Close your eyes and roll your whole body gently. You are now ready to relax deeply.

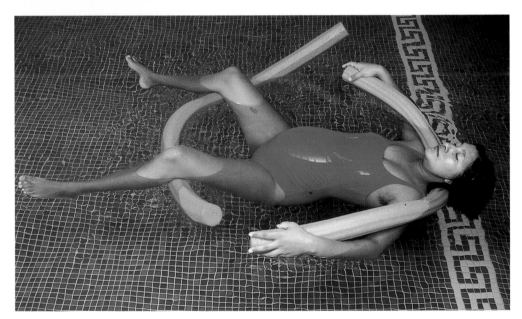

43 With one woggle under the knees and another under your neck

This is perhaps the position in which women can relax the most deeply. Be careful that there is someone watching you in case you completely lose track of time.

◁ **1** Stand in the water with two woggles in front of you. Place the first under your knees as before, then place the other behind your neck. Bring your hands over it loosely on each side to keep it in place. This allows you to stretch yet relax fully.

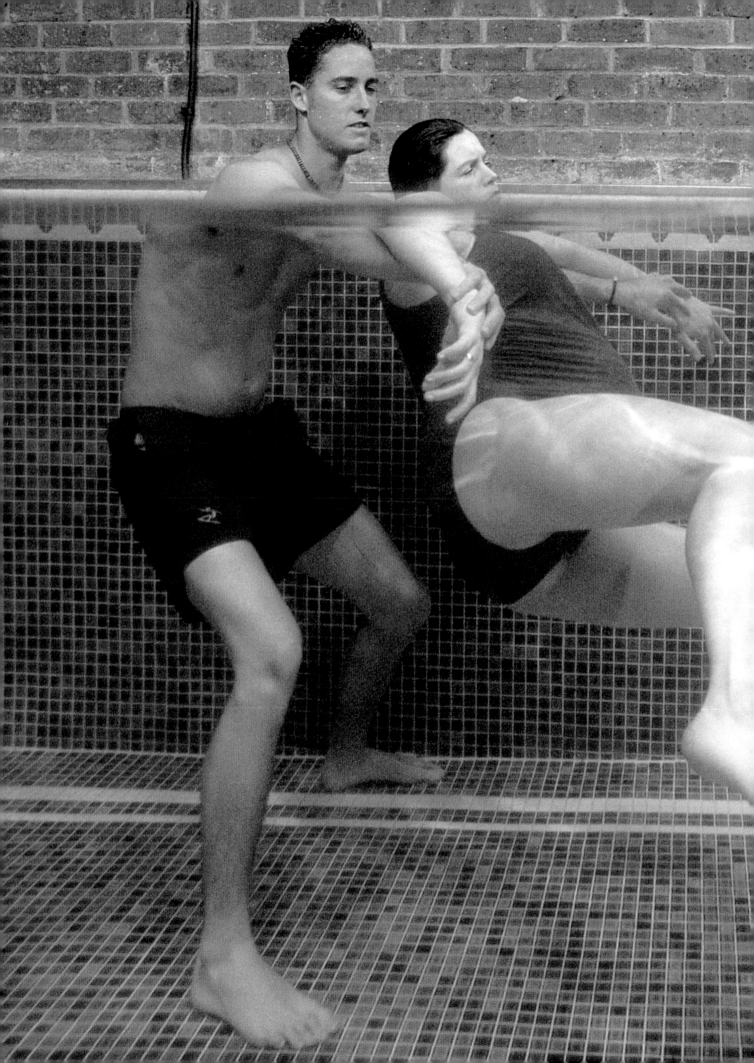

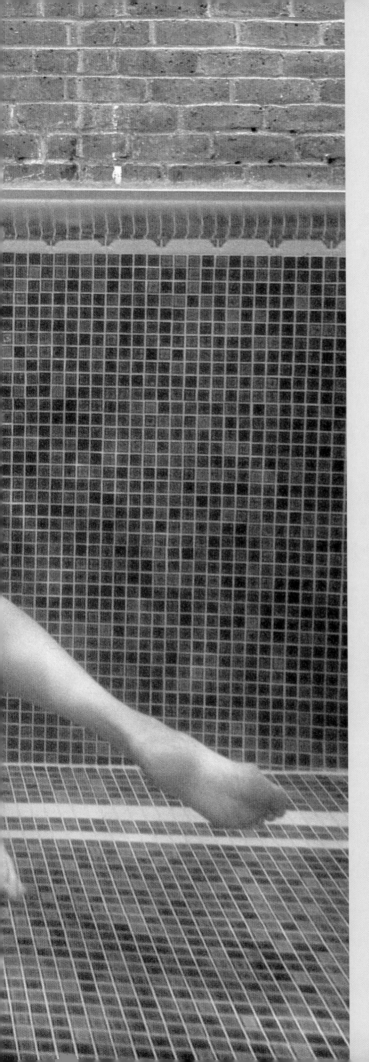

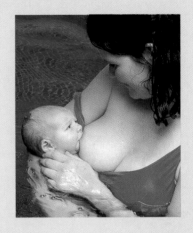

preparing for a
waterbirth

Waterbirth is the renewed discovery of our

ancestral affinity with water applied to birth.

It is a search for comfort in a state that is different

from our normal state of consciousness, where the

need for privacy, intimacy and protection is

intense. Water is gentle on the mother's body and

the baby's entry into the world. Aqua yoga

prepares you for a fuller use of the power of water

to alleviate pain during labour and to ease birth.

The benefits of water in labour and birth

In the last two decades, the use of water to facilitate birth has shifted from the esoteric and the legendary into everyday practice. In the 1980's, experiences of waterbirth fired the enthusiasm of midwives and obstetricians so that women from all walks of life and many nationalities now choose to labour and give birth in water.

Waterbirth is an option that is increasingly available to women in hospitals, homes and birthing centres around the world. Labouring women with low-risk pregnancies, which accounts for the majority of mothers-to-be, can labour in a bath or birthing pool and, in many cases, give birth to their babies in water. The use of water in

labour and birth has now been studied and documented sufficiently to allow emotional views for or against it to be replaced by known facts. Few people still fear that babies may drown when born in water but it is now better known that babies need to be lifted to the surface fairly soon to initiate their first breath, as the blood that continues

A story of a waterbirth: Hester and Bathsheba

Although not many births are as romantic and laid back as the birth of Bathsheba greeted by siblings and the family dogs, Hester's story captures well an experience shared by many women labouring in water. Hester practised yoga to prepare for her three previous births and found the aqua yoga exercises most helpful in making full use of movement and breathing in this birth.

My fourth baby, Bathsheba, was born early in the morning by candlelight into a pool by the fire. Near the beginning the children were still asleep upstairs, my husband was filling the pool and our two midwives arrived and settled calmly on the sofa with the dogs and a pot of tea, not interfering at all.

During early labour I used the pool as a calm, dark space in which to float. It contained me, helped me to focus energy on my mission and connect with the baby. An hour later I was consciously appreciative of the deep heat and massaging effect of the water. The force of contractions felt much less harsh, less frightening in the water. I found this out when I got out for a while to have a walk about and a little dance to speed things up – the strength of the contractions really hit me hard and I got back in quickly.

As the intensity increased, the pool allowed me to move with freedom and vigour. I no longer felt heavy and the water relieved my sciatic pain and stiffness. For the last hour I was moving all the time, keeping the water swooshing around me in a low squat, using a sweeping, arcing movement of the pelvis from side to side, stretching the left leg out far to the side when swinging round to the right and vice versa, hanging on to the side of the pool with both hands. Sometimes I changed the movement to whole circles with the pelvis, a bit like belly-dancing, or I used a swinging backwards and forwards motion. I continually repeated the words, "Open, open" to myself and concentrated all my energy down, breathing long controlled out-breaths through my mouth, sipping water, and really trying to help the baby move down. I was totally driven to keep moving; the more strongly and rhythmically I moved the greater the relief.

I did then completely lose it during transition, and sloshed about wildly like a maniac for a couple of minutes, until Fred caught me from

behind and supported me under the arms for the birth.

I bore down for maybe half a minute and the baby's head slipped out quite easily. I shrieked a bit then and the dogs took the cue and started howling and woke all the neighbours. The baby's body stalled so the midwife reached into the pool and unhooked the cord from behind the baby's neck and brought her gently up into my arms. She lay clean and glowing in the firelight. Her two sisters and brother reached in to stroke her little body, and for the fourth time Fred and I felt humbled before the power of birth, exhausted and thrilled.

Later, the children from next door who had woken to the howling of the dogs came in on their way to school to see the new baby. They saw Bathsheba feeding by the fire, two hours old. The midwives had already gone.

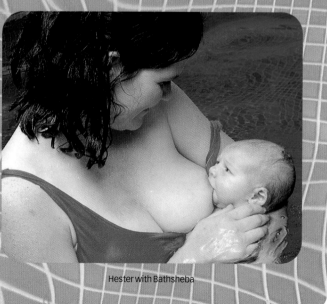

Hester with Bathsheba

flowing through the cord has less oxygen once they have been born. The monitoring of babies born in water has been improved by the use of submersible dopplers. A sound code of practice has been developed for waterbirth both in hospital and at home.

Research has confirmed what midwives have known for generations: water has a relaxing effect on both the mother and her baby. Mothers experience less pain when they labour in water and therefore have less need for pain relief. Water also offers some protection to the perineum in giving birth, although it does not totally eliminate the risk of tearing as early enthusiasts claimed.

The birth experience

For many women who give birth in water, the difference is in the quality of the birth experience. Their statements are difficult to quantify but they share a lyrical, euphoric feeling. Besides comfort and freedom of movement during labour, water gives women the privacy that they need to be able to let go of their fear and enter the mental space in which their labour can progress unhindered. Although it does not eliminate pain, water allows more control over the rhythms of labour.

Many women who want a "natural birth" find that once they are in a hospital environment much of what they have read or learnt is superseded by the protocols and routine practices of the labour ward. Being in water makes it easier to feel centred and in charge. They are then in the best possible state of mind, and body, to meet their new-born babies, perhaps lifting them from the water themselves.

Not all women who plan to have a waterbirth have their babies in water. There are many reasons why a planned waterbirth can become an unplanned dry birth, a practical example being that some babies arrive before the tub is filled up. Babies whose heartbeat slows down during labour may be at risk of oxygen deprivation and may have to enter into the air for greater safety. Equally, many women who have never thought of a waterbirth feel so comfortable labouring in a birthing pool that they just find themselves giving birth in it.

Good for your baby too

This book is concerned with helping mothers to have comfortable pregnancies and easier, less painful births, but birthing in water also has advantages from the baby's point of view. The transition from the womb to water, rather than cold air, is the gentlest possible. Babies are born in a warm environment without the pressures of gravity. Uncurling from the confined space of the womb into the unboundedness of water may create a different quality of birth experience for the baby, and this may have distant repercussions in the make-up of his or her personality. Some people claim that "water babies" have special qualities, being both lively and calm.

Should you not be able to use a pool or even a bathtub during your labour, remember that you can still derive great benefit from water, particularly if you have practised aqua yoga during pregnancy. Even running water from a tap, or a wet sponge on your face, can conjure up the deep relaxation that you have enjoyed in water.

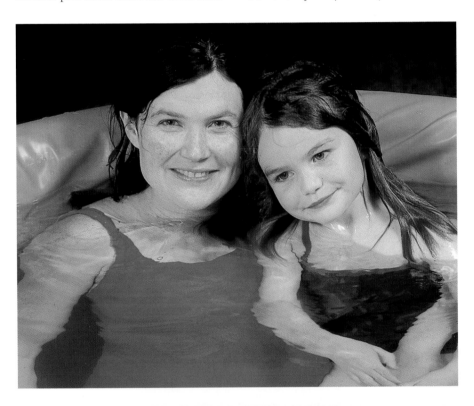

△ When a new baby is about to enter the family, water is also a medium to renew the bonds with your other children.

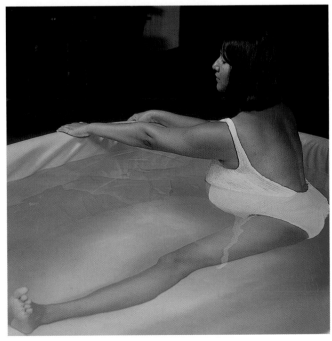

▷ During labour, aqua yoga helps you move around to find the most comfortable positions in the birthing pool.

Opening for birth

Although research has not confirmed that labouring in water makes it easier for the perineum of unprepared women to stretch without tearing, yogic pelvic-floor breathing, to prepare both physically and mentally for this stretching, is equally effective in dry births or waterbirths. Practise it every day during the last six weeks of pregnancy, in the pool, in a birthing pool or simply at home in the bath.

Opening the body for birth is accompanied by a state of being open to what can happen and surrendering to it. You may have prepared well and feel strong, relaxed and confident in yourself, but the journey of your baby's birth can take unexpected courses. Open your mind, letting go of all expectations and plans. Let this birth take its course and be ready to flow with it fully.

If you stay in touch with your baby throughout your labour, it becomes a shared journey and is likely to be a satisfying experience, whatever happens. If the need for intervention arises at any time, remember that breathing and relaxation are invaluable tools. Fear of the unknown is a primary source of muscular tension: so, with each out-breath let go of your fear.

44 Open stands, drops and hip swings

Right up to the day of the birth, open stands and drops help to stretch the lower spine and ease the back. They also facilitate the descent of the baby's head in the pelvis and, after it has become "engaged", promote optimal presentation in an anterior position. This maximizes the space between the coccyx and the pelvic symphysis at the front, so that the baby's head has as much room as possible to rotate forward into the birth passage once the cervix has dilated during labour. Many women feel a need to hang from a support and move their hips before and during labour to achieve this effect. The more these movements are practised during the last six weeks of pregnancy, the greater the chances of an easier and less painful labour.

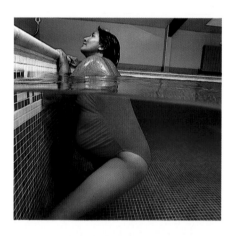

◁ **1** Standing facing the pool wall, inhale. Flex your knees open and let yourself drop – with a straight back – holding on to the bar or the edge of the pool as you exhale slowly. Breathe deeply a couple of times before standing up and letting yourself drop again.

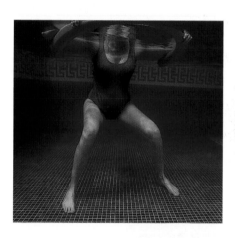

◁ **2** If holding the bar or edge constrains you or is uncomfortable, use a woggle under your arms. Support from the back allows you to drop in a very open semi-squat, while resting your arms on a woggle at the front helps you drop, leaning slightly forward.

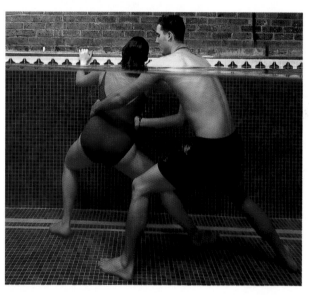

◁ **3** Your partner may hold you while you swing your hips in a semi-squat position, holding on to the bar, the edge of the pool or a woggle in front of you. This helps you to drop the base of your spine lower in the water and open your hips more. You can swing your hips from left to right or complete a circling movement. Keep your neck soft, relaxing your lower jaw.

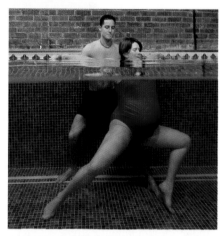

△ **4** The same movements can be done in a more supported way with your partner behind you, holding you with his arms under your arms.

45 Float-drop

While the drops can be done both on the dry land and in water, you can uniquely open your pelvis freely in the water, forgetting gravity and without any pressure on your legs. This is a useful exercise if you would like to have a birth in which you can be absorbed in the process of labour rather than trying to control it. It is also helpful if you wish to have a vaginal delivery after a previous Caesarian section and you need to avoid putting any strain on your scar tissue. Women who wish to have a gentle birth in water can use this exercise to make the most of water as a supportive environment.

▷ **1** Holding on to a woggle in front of you, inhale and let yourself drop gently in the water as you exhale with your legs open and completely relaxed. Continue breathing in this position, half floating, half sinking, feeling every muscle of your pelvis relaxed around your uterus.

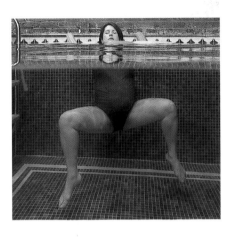

▷ **2** You can also let yourself "float-drop" while being supported by your partner under the arms. He can then swing you from side to side without your legs touching the pool floor. Breathe deeply and enjoy the freedom from gravity in this supported movement, opening your hips as much as possible.

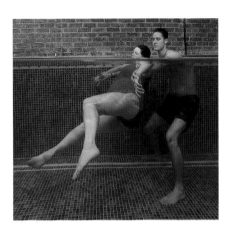

46 Breathe yourself open

The first and most important tool that you will have at your disposal during labour, made even more effective by water, is your breath. As your due date approaches, besides practising aqua breathing you may find the following exercise helpful. Breathe in as you start any of the above positions. Lengthen your out-breath slowly as you lower your body in the water, opening your pelvis wide. You may vocalize the breath if it helps you as a long "Haaaaah" or "Hooooh" sound. As you do this, release any fear that you may have about how your baby is going to be born, the changes that motherhood will bring in your life, the unknown. With your vocal out-breath, calmly empower yourself and feel your energy centre strong and yielding deep inside your abdomen.

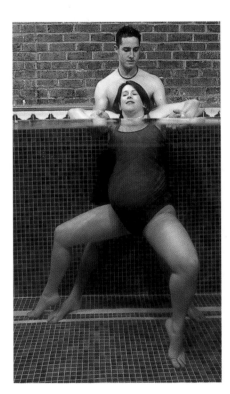

◁ **1** You can practise this breathing on your own or supported by your partner with his arms under your arms while he stands against the pool wall, which is also a possible birth position whether in or out of water.

47 Floating relaxation before birth

As you reach the end of your pregnancy you may wish to practise floating relaxation with your baby's father or your labour partner in anticipation of the birth. Joint floating relaxation can be a powerful way of preparing for birth, which many women recall during labour as a way of centring themselves and keeping a close contact with their baby.

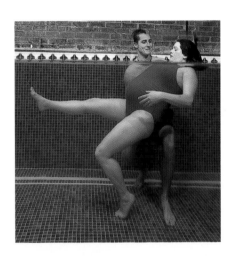

◁ **1** Your partner should place one hand under your lower back and the other at the base of your neck.

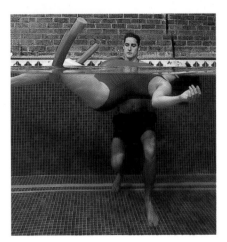

◁ **2** The additional support of a woggle under the knees is often desirable. This takes the strain off the supporter and it also enables both partners to relax together while focusing on the baby between them.

Aqua yoga for labour

When you labour in water, you escape to a peaceful protected world where you can be at one with the rhythm of the contractions and your breathing. Water massages, supports and envelops you in a way that is far removed from being watched in a labour ward. It gives you total privacy and comfort, in your own world with your baby.

Experience gathered from thousands of women by midwives and doctors attending the first International Waterbirth Conference at Wembley, London in 1995 showed that the more the body of a labouring woman is immersed in water, the more effective is the pain relief. Most women did not go underwater during labour, but it helped some to concentrate during painful uterine contractions.

Labouring while in warm water has the advantage of maximizing the supply of rich oxygenated blood to the hard-working uterus in several ways: the muscles that maintain your posture against gravity are supported; major veins and arteries are not obstructed in any position; temperature is even and less blood is diverted to the periphery of the body.

Exercises in the swimming pool or the birthing pool in early labour can help greatly to open the cervix. Short active periods can be alternated with quieter restful ones, during which you can practise visualization techniques or just relax and breathe through your contractions as they come and go.

48 Pelvic rolls and swings in the birthing pool

Rolls and swings increase the pressure of the baby's head in a rhythmical way and involve you actively in the process of making space for your baby to come down into the birth passage.

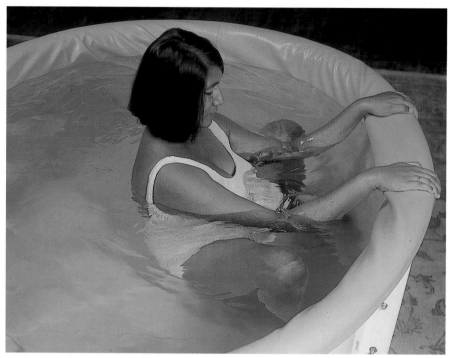

△ **1** Get into a low squatting position, holding on to the edge of the birthing pool.

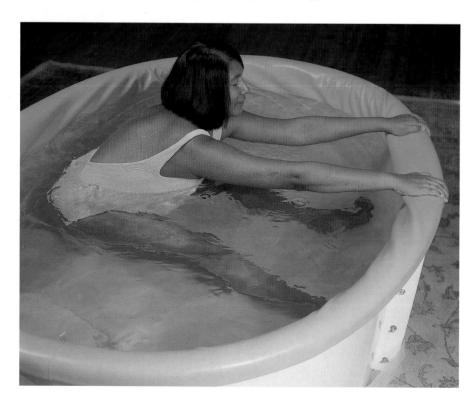

▷ **2** Swing your pelvis forward and back: this will make you bend and stretch your legs in a broad movement. Breathe in as you stretch back, out as you bend forward.

49 Knee-bent variations

These are useful movements which can get a baby "unstuck" from an awkward presentation and help promote stronger labour when contractions become weak during the first stage, as this is usually because the head of the baby is not pressing on the cervix at the best angle.

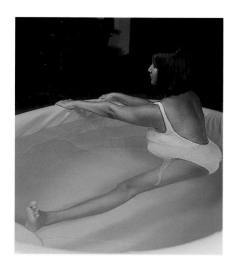

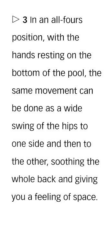

◁ **1** Kneel in the birthing pool, holding the edge in front of you, and straighten one knee and then the other, extending the leg sideways at the bottom of the pool. Breathe deeply, exhaling as you extend either leg to the side, and take your time to feel intuitively which position "opens" you the most.

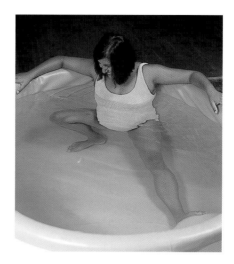

◁ **2** The same leg movement can be practised facing the pool in a squat, with the back against the side of the pool, or in a sitting position. Breathe in the same way.

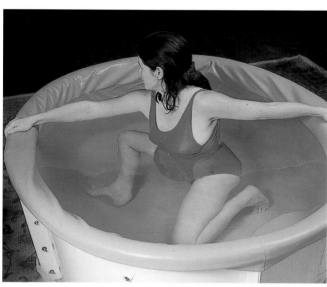

▷ **3** In an all-fours position, with the hands resting on the bottom of the pool, the same movement can be done as a wide swing of the hips to one side and then to the other, soothing the whole back and giving you a feeling of space.

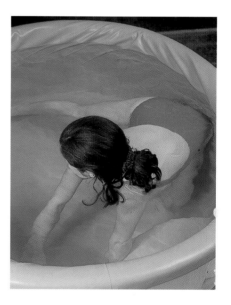

△ **4** With the arms stretching sideways holding on to the opposite edges of the pool, the same alternating leg movement becomes more active and has all the advantages of a deep squat without putting undue pressure on the pubic bones or the perineum. A simultaneous opening of one knee and closing of the other is a very effective way of changing sides. Turn the head in the direction of the raised knee, as in a low-lying archer pose in classic yoga.

▷ **5** Between these movements, take rests in a kneeling position, in which you can also do comforting pelvic rolls now and again. In the early phase of labour, when your contractions are just getting established, you may not mind being visited by your older children if you are having a home birth. Seeing you in the birthing pool involves them in the journey that their little brother or sister has initiated to join their family.

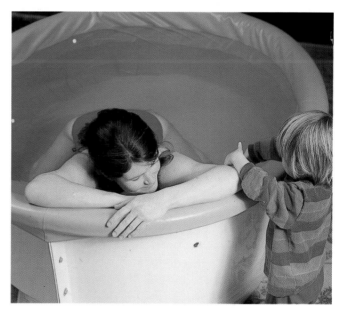

Aqua breathing for waterbirthing

Make it a priority to find a rhythm that will help you move at regular intervals and change position. This will enable you to remain centred and feel the progression of your labour in a positive way. Whether you continue using pelvic rolls and knee-bent movements in the birthing pool or not, try alternating between a forward kneeling position, a lying float and sitting down or, if you are very confident with yoga and breathing into your pelvic floor muscles, squatting. Try different angles, as some may suit you better than others, and then use your favourite positions throughout the first stage of your labour. You may need reminding to move as your labour gets stronger and you become more absorbed in the rhythm of contractions.

Relaxation between contractions

The ability to relax between contractions during labour saves a great deal of energy, which is better used to keep you alert to welcome your baby into the world. It also reduces negative stress, and with it a great part of the discomfort of labour. The only part of your body that needs to contract in labour is the uterus, and active relaxation makes this possible. Sometimes the pain of contractions causes other muscles to tighten up, but a deep exhalation, giving your body, mind and emotions the message to relax, can dissolve all the tension again and again just after it has reached a peak.

During labour the primitive parts of the brain are involved. The safer and more relaxed you feel, the less likely you are to produce "run away from danger" hormones, such as adrenalin, which counteract the "peace and harmony" hormones, such as prolactin, produced when relaxing. Floating relaxation also promotes the production of endorphins, the body's own painkillers, to help you tolerate the physical pain of birth. These hormones also help you to forget about it as soon as it is over.

Using the birthing pool

There is no strict rule about when to get into the water or how long to stay in it during labour. Make sure you keep drinking little sips of water so you do not become dehydrated and that the water temperature remains constant (33–40°C/91.4–104°F in the first stage of labour and 37–37.5°C/98.6–99.5°F during delivery).

When you stand up to get out of the pool in pre-labour or during labour, you may feel dizzy while your circulation readjusts to the effects of gravity. Take it slowly, accepting help to sit on the edge of the pool and swivel your legs over it one at a time. Stand up carefully and take small steps, bending your knees slightly to ease your lower back.

A story of a waterbirth: Alison and Luke

Alison's story illustrates the greater effectiveness of yoga breathing and water in combination during labour. While being accomplished in yoga since her first pregnancy, deep breathing in water proved invaluable to Alison in alleviating a challenging backache in her third birth.

Luke is my third child to have been born in water. Just as the children bring with them their own personalities, each labour has brought new challenges and experiences.

Water has played a significant part throughout all three pregnancies and labours. The stretches and movement that can be achieved in water are quite different from those on land and it has been so reassuring for me to enter a labour knowing that, through yoga, my body has been prepared for the event.

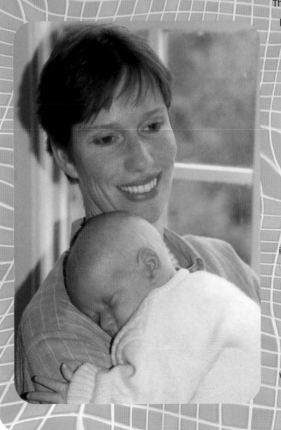

The pool has always given me my own private space – somewhere to let go in and to feel a sense of freedom. In my previous labours I found it much easier to be active and to move around, but this time the contractions came so fast and furiously that I didn't feel like moving at all. However, the simple support that the water offered enabled me to focus on expanding my breathing and channelling the breath in a direction that I had often rehearsed in yoga practice. The pain was intense but for me breathing was the only way of staying grounded and of being able to work with the contractions as they rippled the water around me. Having benefited from Françoise's generous support and wisdom over the last five years, it was particularly special that she was with us to witness Luke's arrival.

50 Breathing through your contractions in water

In any of these positions, each time you feel a wave of contraction starting to tighten the wall of your uterus, exhale to relax and welcome this process, which is squeezing your baby further down to put pressure on your cervix and "open" you further. The more relaxed you are, the more effective each contraction is bound to be. As soon as you feel the completion of the contracting force, often around your navel, exhale again to dispatch this wave and let it follow its course, without engaging in it any longer by feeling pain after it has accomplished its task. This gives you a little extra time to relax and restore your energy before the next contraction comes along, which can be invaluable when they come fast and strong.

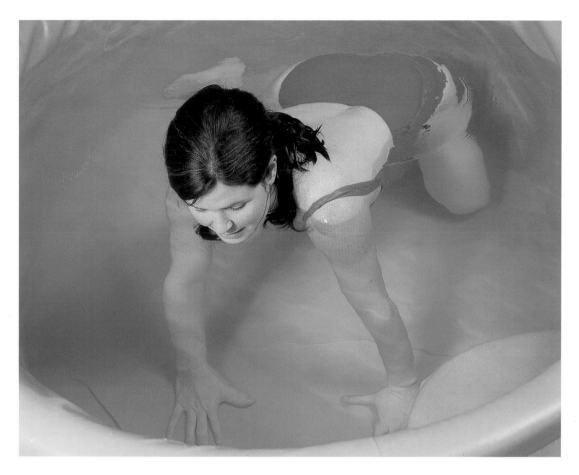

◁ **1** Alternate between positions that suit you throughout your labour. For example, you may find it helpful to kneel upright during a contraction.

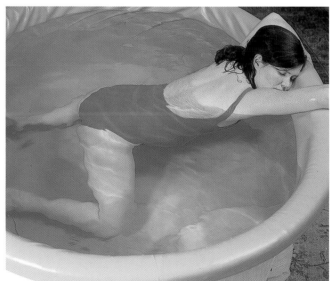

△ **2** As the contraction passes, rest forward on the edge of the pool to start relaxing again.

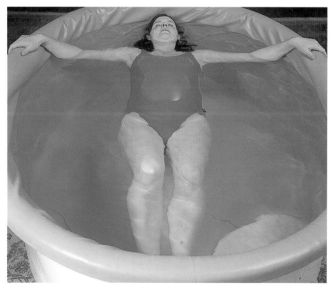

△ **3** You can also rest, breathing quietly and deeply, between contractions by stretching on your back in the water, resting your feet against the opposite wall of the pool while your arms stretch on each side to hold the edges and keep you afloat.

Positions for waterbirthing

Mothers who have moved freely in their late pregnancy and labour tend to move spontaneously into the best possible position for childbirth. While some women feel more open in an upright or slightly backward-leaning position, in a semi-squat or standing, an equal number prefer to lean forward, usually kneeling. Water allows a unique, gravity-free way of giving birth. You can be supported by your birth partner in the tub or support yourself on the edges of the tub and "float" with your bearing-down contractions without having your feet on the bottom of the tub.

If your contractions slow down or seem to peter out when you are fully dilated, recall that traditional midwives call this the "rest and be thankful" stage before bearing down. Standing up in the pool or even getting out for a short walk, interspersed with semi-squats, can do wonders to get you back on track. Keep calm, saving energy.

The time when you are ready for your baby to be born is called the "second stage" of labour, during which more powerful yet not necessarily more painful contractions push your baby through the birth canal (your vagina) and into the outside world. At this time, both the position you are in and your breathing can make a great difference to how you will experience the birth and how your baby will be born. The unfamiliar sensations of second-stage contractions can make you hold back, contracting your buttock muscles involuntarily. Water helps you to let go of fear and open your whole self – body, mind and spirit – to make space for your baby's journey through you.

Without hurrying, allow your body to settle into the most comfortable position to give birth, even if it is not one that you had prepared for.

51 Squat, semi-squat and supported standing

Pace yourself and concentrate on the sensations around your perineum as it stretches to allow for the passage of the baby's head. To avoid tearing, stay as relaxed as possible and if necessary voice your exhalation to slow down the force of the contractions until you feel that the head can make its way through the elastic, expanding tissues of your vagina and perineum. First-time mothers can have the extraordinary experience of accompanying the descent of their baby's head with their breathing, perhaps touching it with one hand just before it appears. If the head is out and the rest of the body still inside you, the shoulders will probably be born with the next contraction, one after the other, before the baby's whole body slips out into the water. In many hospitals, women are now allowed, if not encouraged, to raise their babies out of the water themselves. This can certainly be a peak moment in your life, but something that you can wish for rather than anticipate in expectation.

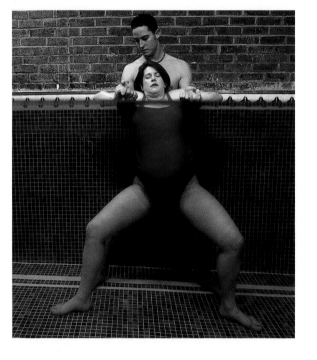

◁ 1 In squatting or semi-squatting positions, make sure that you have a broad, comfortable base with your feet flat on the bottom of the pool. What matters is to create as wide an angle as possible between the base of your spine and your pubic bone so that your baby has plenty of room to move out of your pelvis. Once you start feeling the head in your vagina, focus on lengthening your exhalation at the same time as you feel the strong bearing contractions overwhelming you.

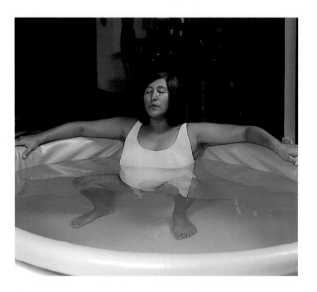

◁ 2 Squatting may not be right for you if you have to exert yourself, or if you have to be on tiptoes or lean forward to sustain the position. In this case, standing half in and half out of the water with your partner supporting you under the arms from behind may be a better option.

52 Kneeling or half kneeling

This position is helpful to relieve back pain caused by the baby's head pressing against your sacroiliac joint. If your baby started labour in a posterior presentation – that is, with his or her back to yours – you may experience less backache with your contractions in this position.

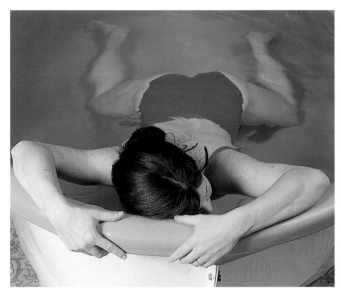

△ **1** This position is about the best you can adopt to relieve back pain and make yourself comfortable, and in water it is particularly effective.

53 Stretch-float

This less common position for waterbirthing suits some women best. Exhaling with contractions, often voicing your exhalation as a chant, scream or grunt, makes this birthing position a very spontaneous one in which you truly surrender to the process and let it take you over.

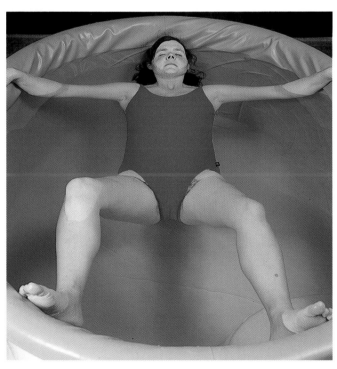

△ **1** In a stretch-float, holding on to the edges of the birthing pool with your head either supported on the edge or just outside the water, you allow the full power of the bearing contractions to push your baby out into the world.

Greeting your baby

Nothing can quite prepare you for the flood of emotions that can overwhelm you when your baby is finally in your arms and here to look at, feel and marvel at as he or she also discovers you. This moment of making contact and welcoming your baby is a precious one indeed, unique to each parent and each birth. Held in the water after starting to breathe in the air, a water baby can adjust gently to being born. It is now common practice to wait until the pulsation stops at the placental end of the cord before cutting it, so that your baby continues to be nourished by the placenta as long as possible. Before your midwife guides you into the third stage of labour, in which you will deliver your placenta, make the most of this initial closeness in the pool which completes your waterbirth. It is now required by many maternity services that mothers get out of the water to expel their placenta so remember that your aqua breathing will also be effective on dry land. After you have rested and your baby has discovered the joy of feeding, it will soon be time to be in the water again. Perhaps a bath with dad too?

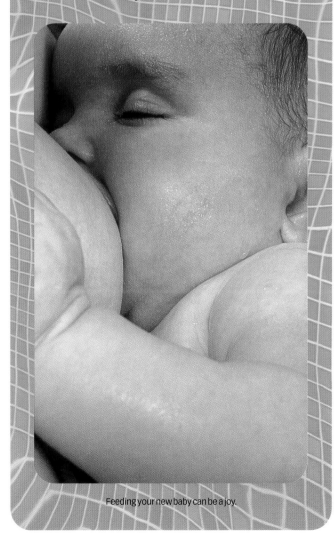

Feeding your new baby can be a joy.

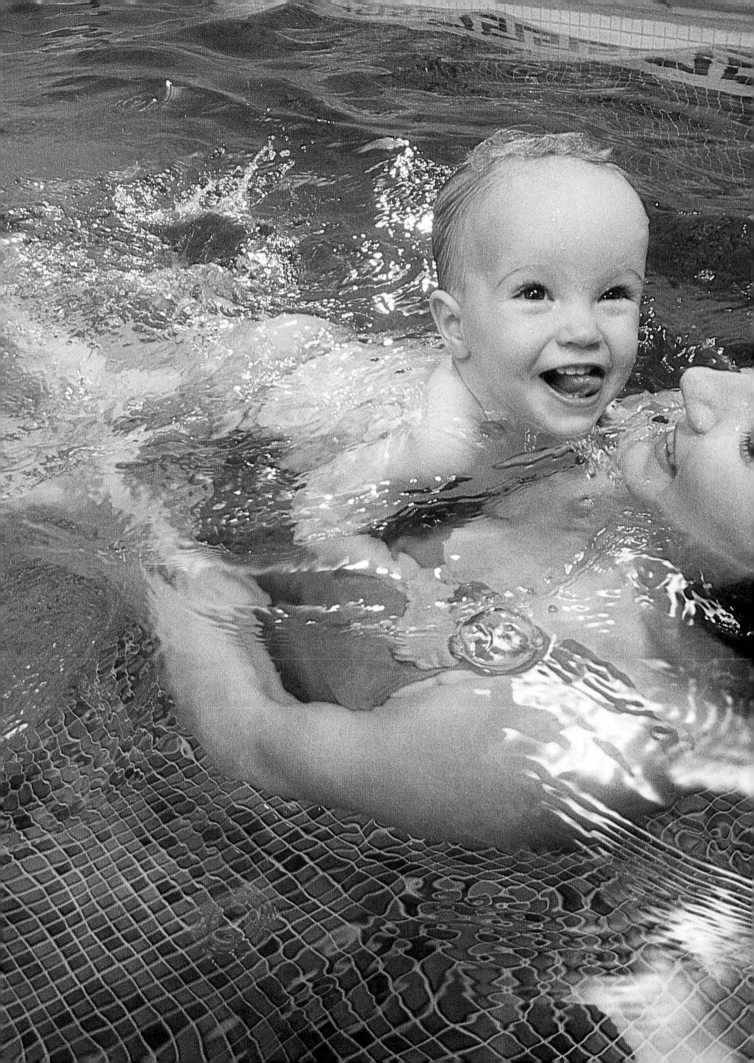

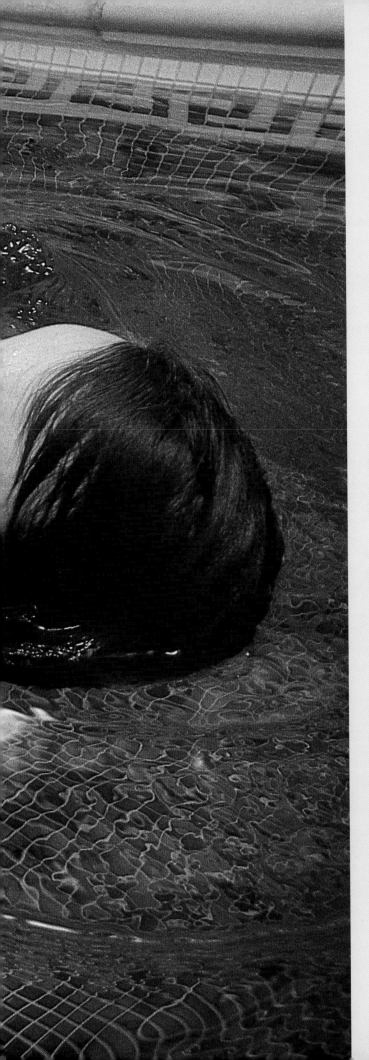

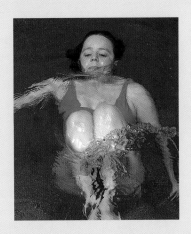

postnatal
aqua yoga and swimming

Now you have done it. You are a mother and here

is your amazing baby. Take time to look back at

what happened during your labour and birth.

Whatever happened, allow feelings of acceptance

to surface and be grateful for the presence of this

child who has come to share your life.

Closing the body

After giving birth, aqua yoga exercises that are the counterpart of antenatal aqua yoga will help you realign and "close" your body, as well as toning and strengthening the muscles of your pelvis and lower back. Water is uniquely healing for the perineum and a good medium in which to tone the pelvic floor muscles. Breathing remains an essential aspect of postnatal aqua yoga.

Rather than aiming simply to "get back to normal", your goal is to create a new strength and stamina which are no less than those of your body before pregnancy but are also enriched by the transformation of birth and – if not yet, before too long – by the fulfilment that being a mother can bring.

Toning with breathing

In the same way that you used your out-breath to "open" your body for birth, relaxing all the muscles of the lower abdomen and pelvic floor, you can now use it in reverse to tone the same muscles. Within a few days, your uterus will have returned to its pre-pregnancy size (an average-size pear). The fitter you are, particularly if you have used deep abdominal breathing in pregnancy, the more elastic the four layers of muscles in your abdomen will be and so more able to tighten, forming a strong and firm abdominal wall. Involving your pelvic floor muscles in aqua breathing will help you achieve thorough and long-lasting results in a relatively short time.

It is best to take advice from your doctor about when you can start going to the pool again, particularly if you have had a Caesarean section. You will benefit from this gentle yet very effective form of exercise earlier than from land-based exercises (these are not advisable until four or five months after the birth).

54 Reverse breathing

The first place to try "reversing" your breathing is in the birthing pool or a bath tub, at home or in the hospital. Either a sitting or a kneeling position, which will allow you to keep your back straight, is suitable.

For a few days after giving birth, take a breath drawing in your abdominal muscles only, without involving your pelvic floor muscles. As you breathe out, draw in these muscles even more. Relax them at the end of your exhalation. It is often a shock to women to discover how soft their abdominal muscles are after having a baby. Do not get discouraged as you can be assured that a steady practice of Reverse Breathing in water will help you tone your abdomen from inside out, from the deepest layer of transverse muscle to the top layers under the skin.

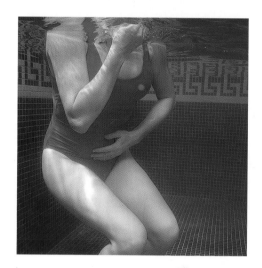

◁ 1 In the pool, it is best to stand with your feet straight under your hips, knees slightly bent, for this breathing to be most effective. Feel the flow of breath having a powerful action on your muscles, to the point that the lower back muscles are also drawn in with your exhalation. Now is time to start lifting the pelvic floor muscles as you inhale and continue lifting them even more as you exhale. Relax them at the end of your exhalation.

55 Cross-kneeling to warrior pose

This exercise can be demanding on new mothers. It tones the oblique abdominal muscles early and effectively after birth, in a way that would not be advisable with land-based exercises until after three months. There is a natural progression from the cross-walks to the classic warrior pose, which you can use now in its aquatic version to stengthen and energize you.

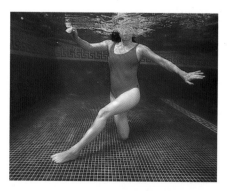

△ 1 Kneel or stand in the pool, depending on the depth of the water, and advance by moving one leg across the other, extending your arms on the surface of the water. If you find it difficult to stride forward, move your crossed front leg back to the centre before moving your other leg forward and across.

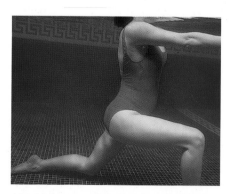

△ 2 Extending your step straight in front of you, bend your front knee so that it is above your foot. Stretch from your back foot, bringing your arms together on the surface of the water in front of you. Breathe in and out in this pose, bringing your back foot forward on the next out-breath. Repeat with the other leg.

Closing the body after birth

After birth, the uterus contracts down to its pre-preganancy size and position within three to six weeks. This process is known as involution. Yoga breathing can ease any discomfort until you have stopped bleeding and feel ready to return to the pool.

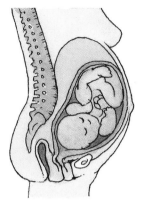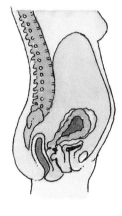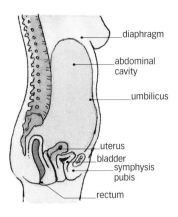

diaphragm

abdominal cavity

umbilicus

uterus
bladder
symphysis pubis

rectum

At the end of pregnancy   Immediately after the birth   6 weeks after the birth

56 Cross-arms

The resistance of the water increases the toning of your arms, upper back and chest muscles in this exercise.

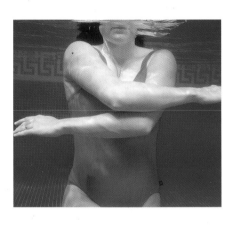

◁ **1** Standing in the water, bring your arms horizontally across your chest with one above the other.

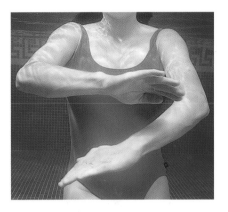

◁ **2** Open them out slightly then bring them back across your chest again, changing the arm that was on the top so that you alternate the crossing of your arms in a vigorous rhythm under water. Breathe in as you extend your arms, out as you cross them.

57 Kneeling close and lift

After months of exercises that helped you to open your pelvis in preparation for birth, kneeling with your knees together is now needed to knit back all the muscles of your abdomen. Reverse Breathing is particularly effective in stretches in which the legs are parallel to each other. The front thigh muscles lengthen and breathing involves both abdominal and back muscles in a tightening effect during the exhalation. In all these exercises make sure that your neck and shoulders are free of tension.

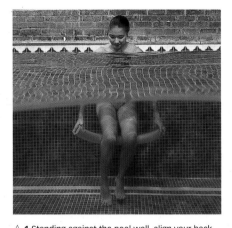

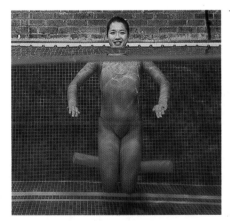

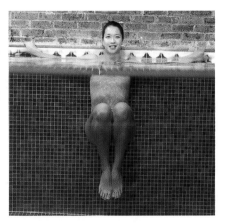

△ **1** Standing against the pool wall, align your back against the wall as you bend your knees, keeping your legs and feet together. You can use a woggle – a half woggle is very comfortable – under the backs of your thighs to help you keep your trunk upright in the water with your knees bent.

△ **2** Your feet can now take off from the pool floor; unexpectedly, you are perfectly stable in this supported upright position which allows you to draw in your abdominal muscles as you practise your Reverse Breathing. The focus is on your hips and legs. You can extend your arms sideways or forward on the surface of the water for additional balance, or hold the edge of the pool behind you.

△ **3** Bring your knees up, holding on to the edge of the pool behind you. Inhale as you lift your knees, keeping them close together, and exhale as slowly as possible with your knees up. Your lower spine will be extended. Doing Reverse Breathing in this pose makes it quite intense for your innermost muscles deep in the pelvis.

Standing aqua stretches

After pregnancy, it is necessary to realign your spine. Standing in the water allows you the maximum stretch between your hip bones and your ribs as you lift your arms above your head. Aqua yoga makes use of deep breathing in relaxed stretches that are easier and safer in water than on land. Your ligaments are still soft and should not be overstretched for at least four months after giving birth.

58 Realigning the spine

Practise these simple standing stretches to lengthen your spinal muscles and breathe deep under your diaphragm where your baby was lying just a few weeks ago.

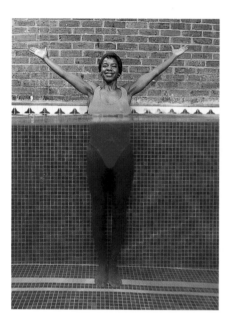

◁ **1** Consciously, with a deep, long breath, close and lengthen your whole body.

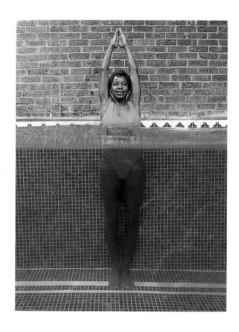

◁ **2** As you stretch your arms above your head, extend to the maximum as you inhale and exhale as deeply as you can. At the end of your exhalation, relax completely and "flop" your arms before you start stretching again on the next in-breath. The fullness of the relaxation is as important as the extension.

59 Overarm stretch

After expanding your breathing capacity during pregnancy, breathing for two, you need to continue using the same muscles which are no longer stretched by your fully grown baby.

▷ **1** You can make the previous stretch more extreme by extending one arm over your head and breathing more intensely in your intercostal muscles: the little muscles between your ribs. Repeat on the other side.

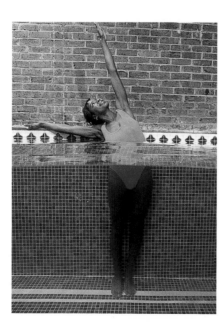

▷ **2** After extending your arm to the maximum above your head, lower it towards your other arm, keeping your chest wide open. Breathe as deeply as possible.

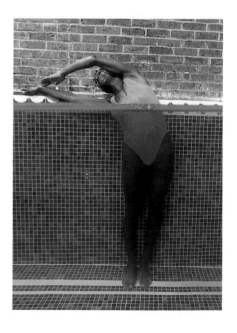

60 Side-stretch

Even more stretch can be achieved by adding a sideways extension to the previous exercise.

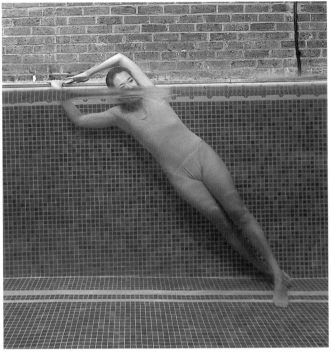

△ 1 With your straight legs together, stretch your whole body in an oblique line, holding on to the bar or pool edge to stabilize yourself with one hand. Stretch first to one side, then to the other, and breathe fully on each side, being aware of creating one long stretch from your feet to your extended hand.

61 Knee-bent stretch

This creates an intense stretch in which you breathe deeply for two or three full cycles before you change legs.

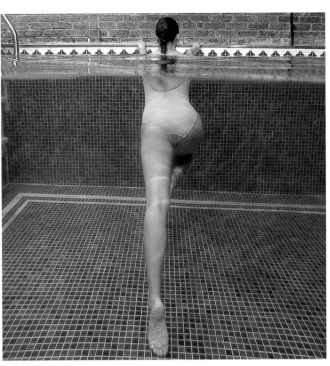

△ 1 Facing the pool wall, take a wide step so that your front foot can rest at the base of the wall. Bend your front knee and lift your foot to bring it onto the knee of your extended back leg.

62 Leg stretch

As you become stronger and fitter, you can practise this classic yoga leg stretch in different ways. At first you may want to rest your leg on the bar, if there is one (the pool edge may be too high). If there is no bar, it may be sufficient to start with to bring your extended leg up, at any height comfortable to you on the wall, while keeping your standing leg bent. Being in water allows a greater stretch than most people can achieve rapidly when doing dry land yoga and strengthens the muscles at the base of the spine that contribute not only to physical fitness but to vital energy in the body.

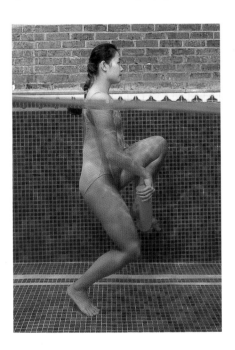

◁ 1 You can use a short woggle to support your leg. Hold both ends and rest your foot in the centre.

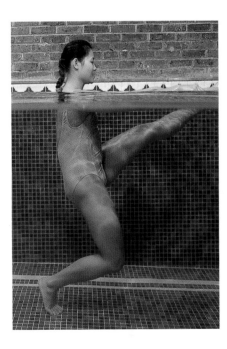

◁ 2 Straighten the leg, bringing your foot up to shoulder height at the surface. Eventually, you will be able to extend both legs, using your stretched legs to pull your back even straighter as you breathe in the pose.

Aqua twists and rolls

These standing twists are a great help in recovering of your waistline, and you will get it back sooner by doing them in the water than you would on dry land. As in all the yoga postures, it is deep breathing that makes the twists effective. The combination of twisting and rolling movements helps to keep your hips supple after pregnancy and prevents postnatal lower backache. If your pool is shallow, you can use kneeling versions of the standing postures. Keep your neck soft and relaxed as you twist.

63 Narrow twists

Both these postures are very helpful if you have split your abdominal muscles in late pregnancy or during birth, and they are recommended if you have had a Caesarean section. Do them facing the wall and holding on to the bar or pool edge, or facing the pool holding on to a woggle or standing freely. Stand with your back straight and your feet together, bending your knees slightly if you need to in order to get a better alignment.

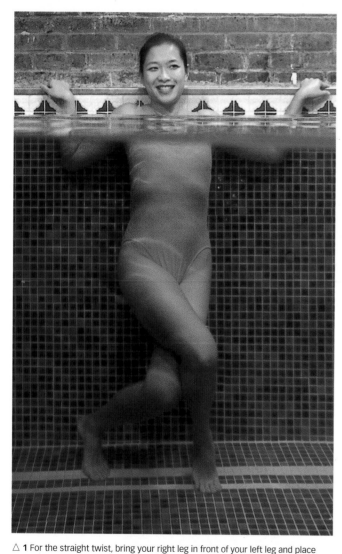

△ **1** For the straight twist, bring your right leg in front of your left leg and place your right foot firmly on the pool floor about 30cm/12in to the far side of your left foot. Keep your hips facing forward. Breathe deeply in the twist a few times, then change legs. If you are kneeling, lift one leg, bring your bent knee in front of the knee resting on the pool floor and place your foot firmly to the outside of that knee, breathing deeply.

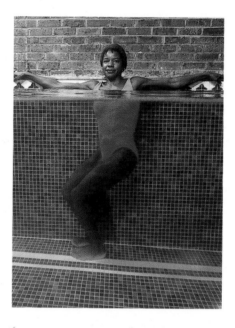

◁ **2** The sideways version gives a more extreme stretch which does not involve opening your hips. Turn both feet to the same side while keeping your trunk facing forward. Breathe deeply in this twist. Repeat on the other side.

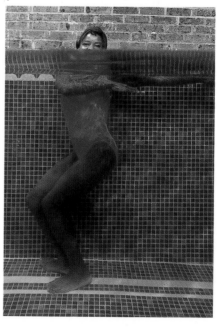

◁ **3** If you are standing or kneeling without support, extend both arms to the opposite side to increase the twisting movement through the whole of your back.

64 Wide twist

For this twist, hold on to the bar or edge if you face the wall; hold a woggle or stand freely if you face the pool. Start from a standing position with your feet wide apart.

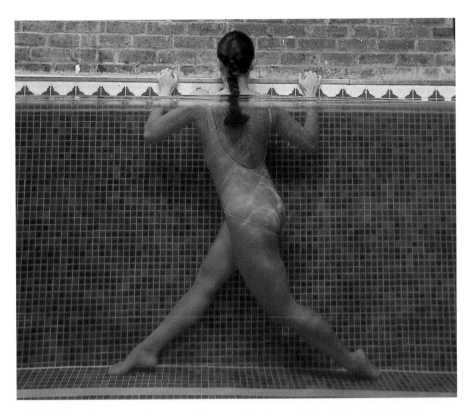

◁ **1** Scissor your legs one in front of the other. Extend your front foot sideways as far as you comfortably can in order to increase the twisting stretch and breathe deeply in this posture a few times. Gradually, both shoulders will become aligned as you face the wall. Let your head follow the extension of your spine naturally. Don't force it.

▽ **2** Change legs and repeat. If you wish to make the posture more dynamic, you can jump and scissor your legs one way and then the other, inhaling as you change sides and exhaling as you stretch down.

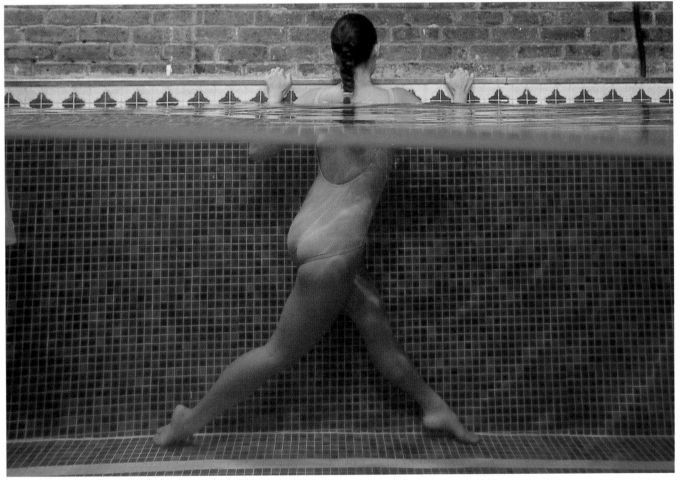

65 Twist-roll-bend

This is a soothing movement for the lower back which also tones the abdominal muscles as you breathe rhythmically with the roll. It can be done facing the wall or the pool, supporting your arms on the bar or on a woggle. If you are in a shallow pool, you can "twist-roll-bend" in a sitting position with your back straight, supporting your arms on a woggle and moving your knees to one side.

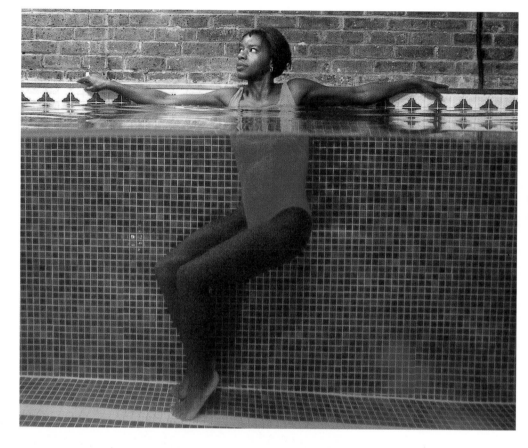

▷ **1** Start from a standing position with your feet together. Keeping your back straight, bend your knees slightly and turn them to one side, creating a gentle twist. Then roll your knees in small circles on that side, bending more as you come to the centre. Make it a fairly energetic movement, breathing in a rhythm that helps you twist further. Repeat on the other side.

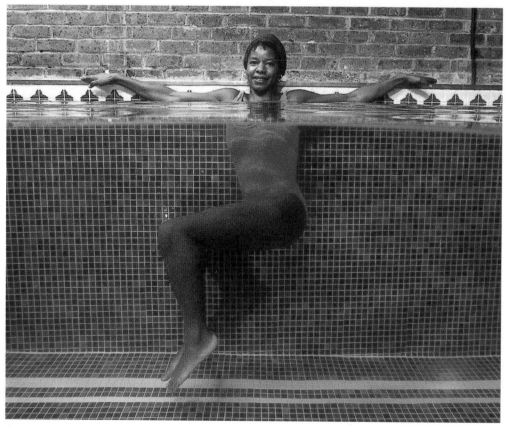

◁ **2** Once you are familiar with the "twist-roll-bend" movement, you can practise it with your feet off the pool floor and your knees up in the water. Now the movement comes from your hips and lower back and you can breathe more deeply in your lower abdomen. It is however more strenuous and may not be suitable for women who have had a Caesarean section in the first three to four months after giving birth.

66 Eagle pose

This is one of the most "closing" classic postures in hatha yoga. It is also beneficial for centring and helps you focus your attention. For all three reasons, it is an excellent pose to practise after giving birth. Even if you are already familiar with yoga, you may find this pose easier in the water than on land after opening your body in childbirth. You can get into the posture progressively, starting with the legs and arms separately before binding both at the same time, and you can use the pool wall as a support behind you to help you balance. You may find that this pose, which is perhaps the one that differs most from all the yoga you have practised during pregnancy, will help you "close" your body and gradually encourage you to turn your attention outward again as your baby is growing.

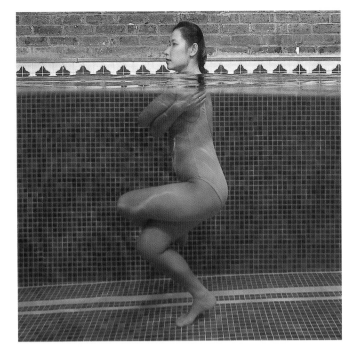

▷ **1** Stand with your back straight and your knees slightly bent. Lift one leg and bring it over your other leg, binding your foot behind it as high as you find comfortable between the ankle and the knee. Feel the closing twist of your hips and breathe as deeply as possible for a minute or two. Then unfold your legs, returning to a standing position, and change sides.

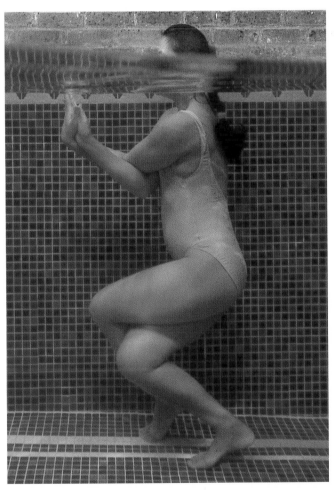

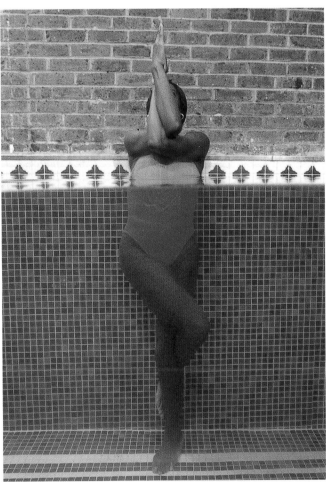

△ **2** In the same standing position, open your arms wide and bring your right arm over your left arm, crossing your arms at the elbows if possible. Then pull your right forearm to the right and bring your right hand forward to meet your open left hand. At first this may be challenging, but with practice your hands will join each other more easily. Breathe deeply in the base of your lungs for a minute or two before unfolding your arms. Change sides and repeat with your left arm over your right arm. This is a powerful toner for the muscles of the upper arms.

△ **3** When you are ready to try the full pose, bring your right leg and right arm over your left leg and left arm and bind them as described in the previous steps. Breathe intensely in the pose, involving your abdominal muscles and all your back muscles in your breathing. In accordance with the classic Eagle pose, select a point in front of you at eye level and concentrate your gaze on this point, centring yourself at the same time and using both breathing and alignment to close your body.

Swimmers' bends and stretches

If you are a swimmer, after stretching with standing poses in the water to elongate your spine and close your pelvis, you can now stretch while swimming to realign your body and remodel your figure after giving birth. Swimming helps you achieve further stretching with twists, bends and rolls in fluid movements which are all the more effective if you do them very slowly and thoroughly.

67 Front and back stretch

Enjoy a plain stretch of your arms and legs together, extending your whole body on your front and then on your back. It is your breathing that makes this stretch tone you, so make sure that you extend more each time you exhale, three to four times on each side. If you are familiar with the start of backstroke swimming from the wall, with your knees bent high, or if you practised the back arch in yoga before your pregnancy, you can also use this movement in water as a safe and gentle postnatal stretch.

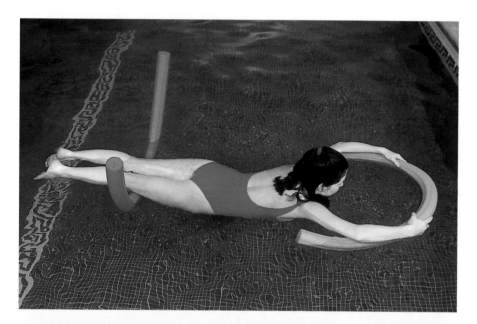

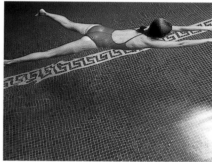

◁ **1** If you are not a confident swimmer, you may wish to use woggles to stretch.

△ **2** If you are a swimmer, extend your arms and legs freely as close to the surface as you can.

◁ **3** Stretch one side and then the other, keeping your arms and legs parallel and, if possible, together, and breathing deeply in your waist area.

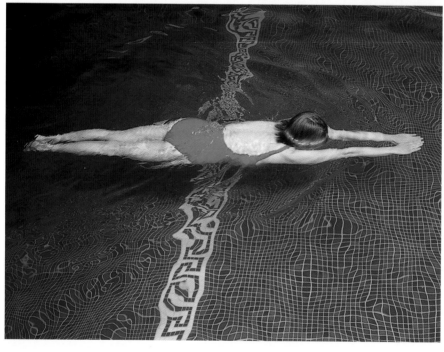

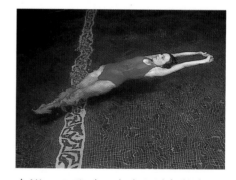

△ **4** You can extend your back stretch further into a back arch. Start by facing the wall with your knees bent, push yourself off the wall and open your front ribs, letting your head and arms follow the movement of your spine.

68 Screw stretch

You can do this movement supporting yourself on a bar at the side of the pool, but it can also be done with a woggle or freely if you are a confident swimmer. Find a rhythm of breathing that suits you in this movement and make sure you roll equally in both directions. The combined rolling and stretching may give you a feeling of physical freedom.

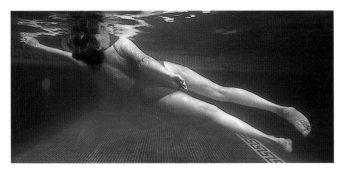

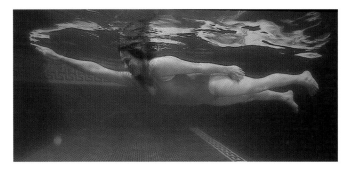

△ **1** In a continuous movement, roll over in the water, extending your right arm and right leg over your left arm and left leg. This combines an extreme stretch with a twisting movement of your whole body.

△ **2** Inevitably, you will have your face in the water some of the time, so you may avoid this movement if you would rather not be under water.

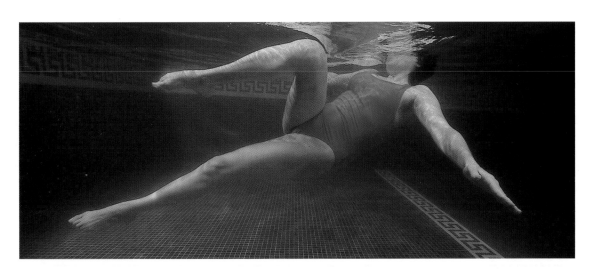

◁ **3** As you become familiar with this rolling twist, you can intensify its "screwing" action by bending the leg that you twist over, while the other leg continues to extend in a relaxed way as you roll.

69 Bend-stretch

This is an expanded, combined version of standing aqua stretches. It elongates the spine and tones the lower back and abdominal muscles together, while stretching the upper back and arms as well. While in pregnancy your aim was to open your knees and hips wide in this movement, now in its postnatal version the emphasis is on the closing of the hips and the stretch.

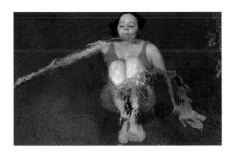

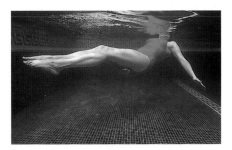

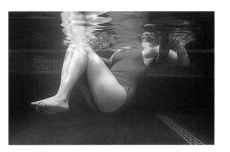

△ **1** Lie on your back in the water with your arms outstretched. Hold on to a bar or a woggle if necessary. Inhale, then, with your legs together, bring your knees as close as you can to your abdomen as you exhale. Stretch again as you inhale and continue alternate stretches and bends for four or five cycles of breathing.

△ **2** In the same starting position, inhale, bring your knees close together then stretch your legs and your whole body as you exhale. Find a steady rhythm which allows you to stretch fully with the flow of the breath. The sculling movement of your arms in and out is an intense exercise in itself.

△ **3** Bend your knees and allow your thighs and trunk to stretch as your knees drop in the water. If you are in a shallow pool, you may find yourself kneeling on the pool floor. Swing your legs back towards your arms and then forwards, raising them to the surface as much as you can. Do not force this bending and stretching movement but let it be fluent even if you find that it is very small to start with.

Swimmers' twists and bends

These twists and bends build on the Bend-stretches (69), including further twisting movements of the whole body in the water. They are quite strenuous and you may not feel ready to start doing them until your baby is five or six months old. Never force yourself. Although you are unlikely to strain your muscles in the water, you can deplete your energy if your practice exceeds your current level of fitness. Every woman is unique and experiences the postnatal period in a different way that she cannot always predict from her degree of fitness before or during pregnancy. Reassure yourself that you can take the time you need to tone your body in depth and always practise under your limit rather than to your limit. Take your time and enjoy each pose fully.

70 Extended twist

As you extend your legs in this position, your arms stretch too so that you get an intense stretch of your whole body in a vigorous rhythmical movement. The higher you bring your knees up before rolling them to the side, the more extended the twist as you then stretch your legs. To start, lie on your back in the water, holding on to a bar or woggle if necessary, with your arms extended.

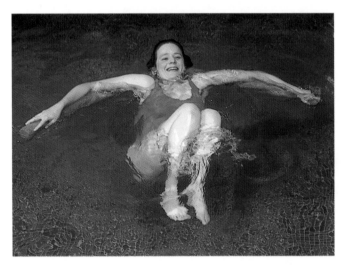

△ **1** At first you can warm up by bending your knees to one side, stretching your legs and then bending your knees to the other side, bringing them as far up as possible each time. Inhale as you stretch, exhale as you bend your knees up.

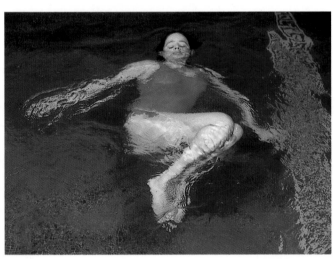

△ **2** Then continue with an expanded version of the standing Twist-roll-bend (65), alternately bending and circling your knees to one side, then extending your legs on the surface of the water before bending and circling your knees on the other side, breathing deeply throughout the movement, keeping your neck soft.

▷ **3** A more advanced version of this exercise is to roll over as your knees drop to the side, bringing your arm over to reach the bar or woggle so that you are now facing down and stretching on your front. Then bring your bent knees together under your body and turn them to the opposite side, opening your arm and lifting it to reach the bar or woggle so that you find yourself on your back once again. Roll three or four times in this way with a steady flow of your breath, enjoying a complete movement that involves all your spinal and abdominal muscles at once.

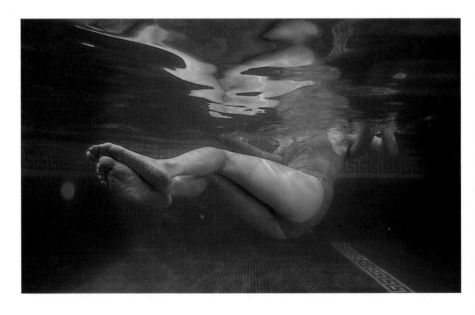

71 Snake bend

The gentle bend of your back in this pose is soothing after stretches and twists, and you can use it as a counterpose and a rest. You can also, however, make it into a vigorous pose in its own right, using the movement of your shoulders and hips to propel yourself. You can practise the snake bend either with your head in water or above the surface. Whether you are a confident swimmer or not, you may wish to use a woggle at first to achieve a very relaxed stretch.

Deep breathing in this exercise makes it a powerful waist trimmer as you involve both your intercostal and dorsal muscles in the stretch. With each exhalation, you can tone the area between your ribs and your hip bones, with visible results after a few sessions at the pool.

▽ **1** Start from a standing position and align your body on the surface of the water, floating face down. If you like, you can use a woggle to support your arms and keep your head above water and another to support your legs and help keep your back straight. Extend one side of your trunk at a time, elongating all the muscles.

▽ **2** Turn your head to the other side and stretch more, breathing as deeply as you can and keeping your bending side relaxed.

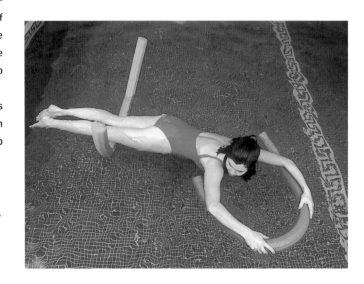

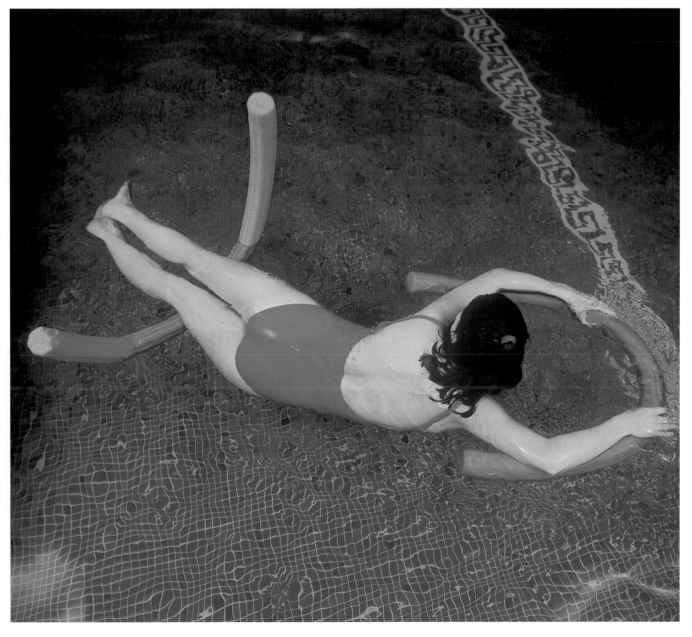

Postnatal front crawl

If breaststroke and its leg movements were ideal to open the hips in pregnancy, front crawl is best to elongate the spine and tone the abdominal muscles of new mothers, whatever their birth experience has been. Front crawl is suitable for those who have had a Caesarean section if it is practised as aqua yoga, using the flow of breath combined with slow motion. This stroke helps new mothers to maintain the expanded breathing they have gained if they have done aqua yoga in pregnancy, and use it now to create new strength and stamina. For those starting aqua yoga postnatally, the goal is to use the full flow of the breath with the swimming movement and gain as much extension as possible with each stroke, rather than aiming at a speedy movement. This is a good stroke for reshaping your buttocks and legs after pregnancy and for elongating your whole body.

72 Leg movement only

The leg movement of front crawl is most effective to tone the abdominal muscles postnatally if it is done in an aqua yoga way: that is, with the legs extended yet relaxed, and the alternate "kicking" motion of the feet coming from the ankles, with the feet remaining soft and relaxed like flippers throughout the movement. In this way the stretch extends via the legs to the abdominal muscles and the deeper muscles of the lower back that control leg movements. Combined with deep breathing, this movement involves and tones the whole body including the legs, trunk and arms.

It can be practised holding on to a bar or to the pool edge, which makes the kicking action more energetic, but it is best done holding on to a float or a woggle as it is less likely to be mechanical and stretches the whole body in movement. Make sure that your arms are fully stretched ahead of you, whatever you are holding on to.

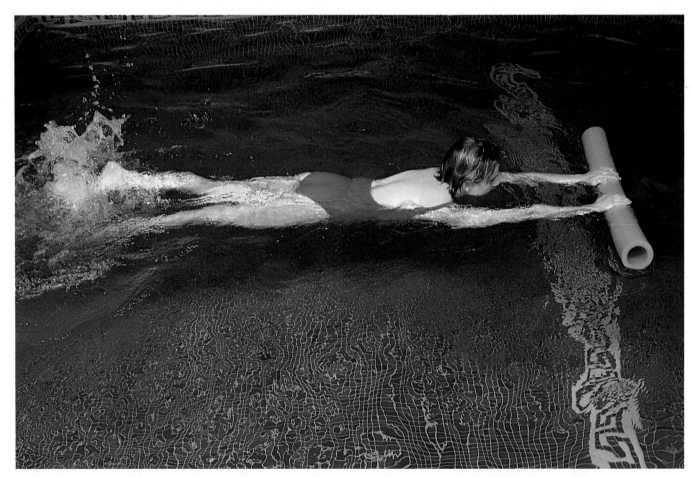

△ **1** Practise relaxing your legs more and more in the kicking action until you feel the movement extending your leg from the hip to your toes, keeping your ankles floppy. Experiment with various amplitudes of movement, from very small kicks just under the surface to a wider movement of your legs under water before your feet splash slightly on the surface.

73 Arm movement only

To practise the arm movement, support your legs so that they remain motionless, with your feet under a bar, or on top of a woggle. You may also place a woggle under your thighs for more support. The movement is very vigorous if you have your feet under a bar but you will almost inevitably have your face in the water. With your feet on a woggle, you can keep your face above the surface, although your body is better aligned if the water comes to your forehead. Turn your face towards your arm to inhale, then exhale in the water as you complete your arm movement.

You make this practice "aqua yoga" by focusing on the extension of each arm, which should be as slow and complete as possible, accompanied by a long exhalation. Inhale on one side each time you extend your arm back on this side, but change sides regularly to avoid getting used to breathing always on the same side.

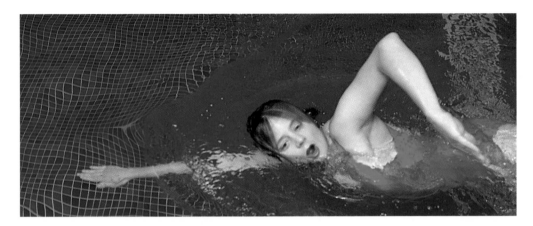

◁ **1** Extend one arm behind you in a sweeping movement and bring it forward as far as you can alongside your ear, turning your hand outwards as it reaches the water. At the same time, start extending the other arm back with the same movement, so that you pull the water vigorously with each arm alternately to the side before extending it ahead.

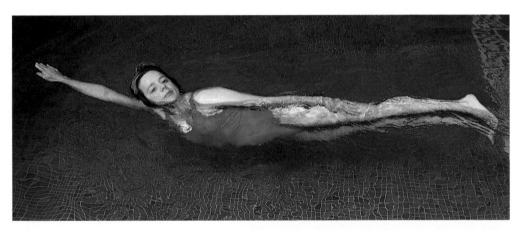

◁ **2** If you are a confident crawl swimmer, keep your feet together and let them trail in a relaxed way close to the surface while you practise this arm movement as slowly as possible, extending your whole body with the stretch and concentrating on the flow of the breath.

74 Front crawl stretch

After practising the leg and arm movements of front crawl separately, this stroke is easier to do in an aqua yoga way, with a slow and thorough extension of each side of the body in turn. There are several possible breathing rhythms you can adopt with this stroke. You can continue to expand your breathing capacity by inhaling on each second, third or fourth arm movement, extending your exhalation more and more.

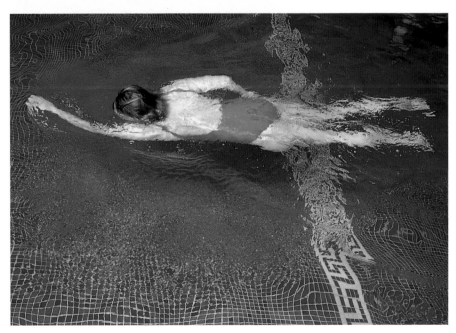

▷ **1** Stretch each arm to the fingertips and use a very relaxed propelling motion of the legs and feet.

Postnatal back crawl

Back crawl is probably the best postnatal stroke. It suits most women as it does not involve having your face in the water as front crawl does. It has a direct and effective action on the abdominal muscles, thighs and buttocks. It can be practised effectively with supports even if you are not a confident swimmer, and you may get great satisfaction improving your performance rapidly by practising the leg and arm movements separately, making it aqua yoga rather than simply a swimming stroke.

A good alignment of the whole body, particularly of your head, neck and back, is essential to achieve both a relaxed stretch and optimum balance when the leg kick and the alternating arm pull are combined. The more relaxed you are in the movement then the easier it is to gain a steady balance and a fluent arm movement. Give priority to breathing in both separate leg and arm movements. In the actual stroke, explore rhythms that give you the greatest free-flowing mobility.

75 Leg movement only

If you start doing this leg movement less than four months after the birth, you may find it difficult to bring your feet to the surface. Persevere and try to keep your movement small, which is a challenge after your hips have become used to wide movements in late pregnancy. It is also important to keep your knees straight so that the legs are stretched yet relaxed at the same time. If you find that you cannot do this leg movement without bending your knees a little, keep practising and concentrate on the motions of your ankles and feet. Gradually, you will find that you become able to keep your legs extended while your feet make a small splash on the surface of the water.

Practise the movement holding on to a bar or a woggle or, if you need more support, use one or two woggles under your arms. You can also hold a float under your head as if it were a pillow. Alternatively, you can hold one or two floats on your abdomen with your hands crossed on top.

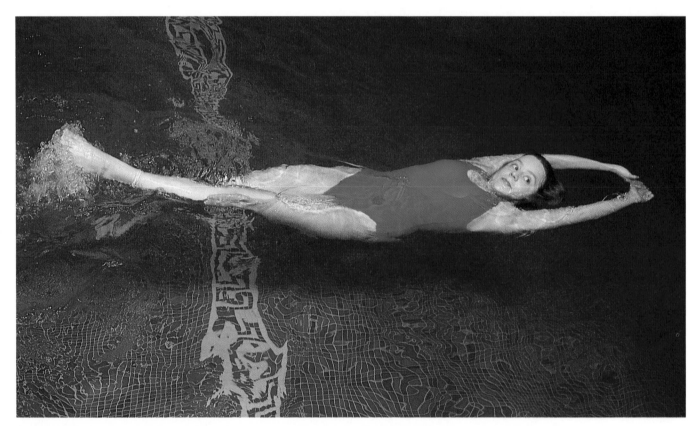

△ 1 Lie on your back in the water with your arms stretched out behind your head. Scissor your legs alternately in the water with a relaxed kicking motion of your feet, legs and ankles, remaining relaxed throughout. Breathe deeply in the movement, extending your exhalations as long as possible. Be aware of the effect of your leg kick on your abdominal muscles and modify it as the muscles that surround your uterus tone again month by month.

76 Arm movement only

In this exercise priority is given to the opening of the chest and the use of the muscles under your ribcage in order to achieve a maximum stretch. Whether you are an accomplished swimmer or not, practising the arm movement of back crawl in this way will stretch each side of your whole body as you swim on your back.

If you are an experienced swimmer, you can do the arm movement in the aqua yoga way, keeping your feet together close to the surface. There is no need to tie your feet together and you may get a better stretch without using a foam block between your feet.

You can also practise with your feet under a bar or with the back of your legs resting on a short woggle. A bar allows more stability and vigorous movement, while the woggle enables you to stretch more slowly and lightly. It is important that you extend your arms and hands in a line, all the way to the fingertips. Stretch to the tip of your middle finger. Find a rhythm of breathing that suits you, every two to four movements according to your capacity.

77 Back crawl stretch

You can now combine the leg and arm movements in the stroke, but if you find that you remain relaxed and aligned in the separate movements but tense up when combining them in the stroke, it is preferable to continue practising the leg and arm movements separately. The more you stretch, the better you will eventually swim, besides gaining stamina and developing strong yet graceful muscles. Swimming in the slow lane, you will soon discover that you cover greater distances with a remarkable economy of movement, making full use of both the relaxed stretch in your arms and legs and your deep breathing.

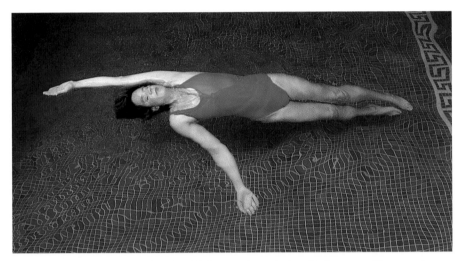

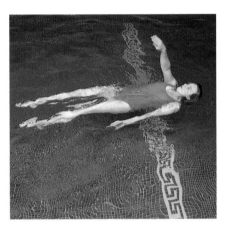

△ **1** Raise one arm with the palm of your hand facing towards your body and in the course of the upward movement, turn your hand so that it faces outwards. Do this with a deep inhalation that opens your chest and make sure that your arm is as close to your ear as you can have it before you extend it behind you as far back as you can. By the time your hand approaches the water behind you, your arm is beginning its oblique pulling that propels you in the stroke. At the same time the other arm comes up with the same circular movement. Keep your chin tucked in so that you are able to see the opposite side of the pool, if not your own feet.

△ **1** Give priority to your alignment and the alternate full stretching of your arms along your ears and back. Keep swimming very slowly, breathing as fully as possible and lengthening your exhalation gradually.

78 Rolling back crawl/front crawl

If you enjoy performing the Screw Stretch (68) you may wish to roll and stretch from front crawl to back crawl. If you do it very slowly and breathe deeply as you stretch to your maximum, you are unlikely to get dizzy and you will probably enjoy the rolling motion of this twin stroke.

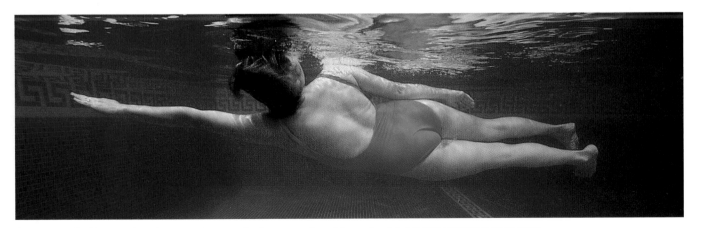

△ **1** Turn your shoulders over in each movement as you extend your arms alternately, one forward as in front crawl and then the other backward as in back crawl.

Postnatal dolphin dives

During pregnancy, dolphin dives are a way of feeling weightless with a broad undulating movement in the water. Indeed, close to the birth, it is even difficult sometimes to go under, and the most pleasant part of the dive is the middle part, before floating back up. After birth, the situation changes and you can enjoy streamlining your body again in the dives, stretching fully in a more vigorous movement that alternates bending and arching your middle spine. Practising these dives helps your back to gradually regain or acquire the flipping motion of the dolphin stroke, which is a perfect toner for back, abdominal and thigh muscles together.

79 Dolphin dives

The alternate bending and arching of your back in succession enables you to take these dives with an even, flowing movement as you practise. Enjoy coming back towards the surface with a greater stretch which may remind you of the stretch-breathing you practised in late pregnancy, although now the feeling you have is quite different.

As you run out of your out-breath, with your arms fully extended in front of you, keep stretching into your waist area. The emphasis is now on "stretch-relaxing" to get further stretch, rather than merely on relaxing as it was before birth. If you swim butterfly stroke, you may wish to first recover the movement of your lower back with dolphin dives before practising the leg movement of the butterfly stroke, holding on to a board with your extended arms.

Diving from the edge of the pool or from diving boards can be uncomfortable for some time after giving birth unless you are an experienced diver. Dolphin dives allow you to get ready for diving again in a gentle way. Once your baby is over four or five months, you can combine them with a Back Stretch (67), arching your back as you dive with your arms extended back.

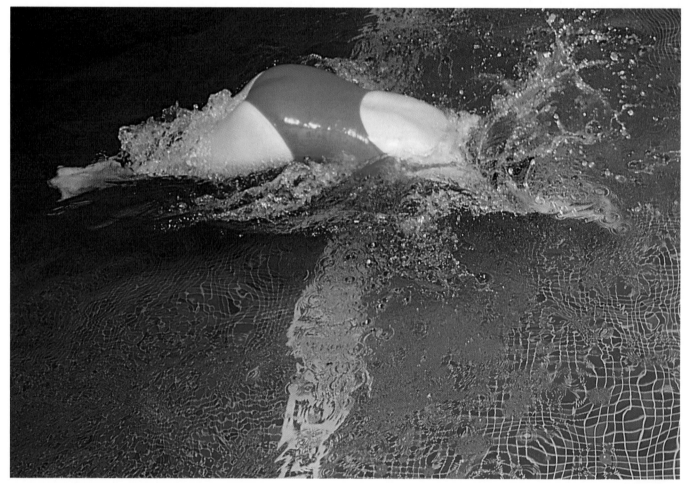

△ **1** Start standing free in the pool. Bend your knees and raise your arms over your head very straight as you inhale. Bend over towards the water and, as you get near, spring on your legs to take a small dive.

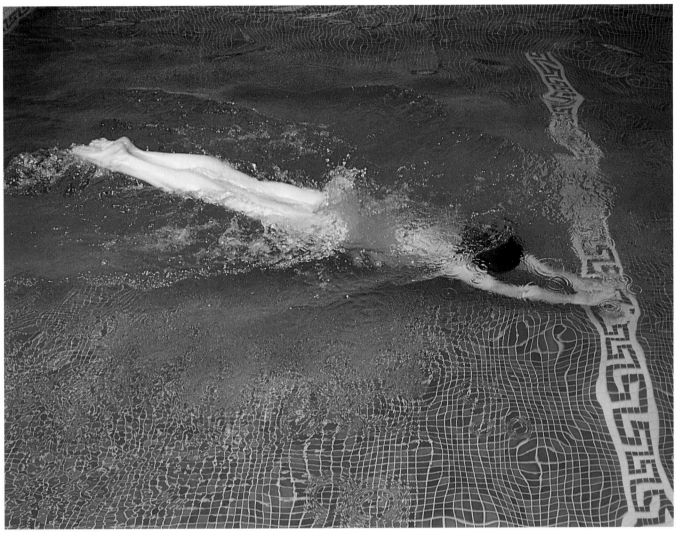

△ **2** As soon as you go under, stretch your lower back and open your chest.

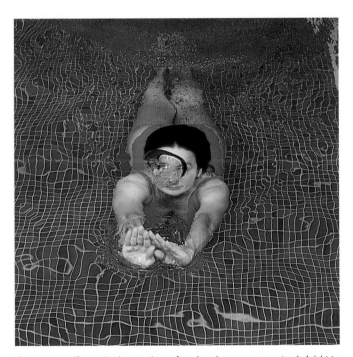

△ **3** Let yourself come back up to the surface, keeping your arms extended right to the end of your exhalation. Then spring again on to your feet, inhale as you stretch and take another dive forward.

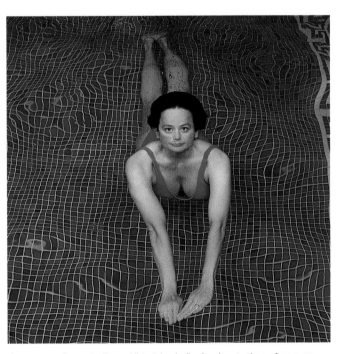

△ **4** You can choose to dive and "stretch-relax" quite close to the surface or go deeper, right to the bottom of the pool, wherever it feels best for you. You can also practise dolphin flips holding on to a board.

Involving your baby

You can involve your baby in your postnatal aqua yoga practice practically from birth at home in your family bath. Many parents prefer to wait until their babies have been immunized before taking them to a public pool. Your baby is protected from polio with the first vaccine, but always follow your doctor's advice about full protection and be aware of your responsibility when you take a young baby to a pool. You are the best person to decide when to take your baby to the pool for the first time. If you have access to a warm, clean pool, the earlier the better.

It is enjoyable to swim with your baby, both as a continuation of your antenatal aqua yoga and because it is also the best introduction to swimming for your child. This section offers suggestions for mothers who are confident in the water. The main challenge is to stay relaxed: if your baby falls off your body into the water, gently pick him or her up and continue. Your baby is likely to be more affected by your agitation than by being immersed. Many babies do not cry at all when they "go under". It is, however, a good idea to have someone with

you when you take your baby to a pool, at least for the first few visits until you gain confidence. If your baby's first introduction to the pool is not a happy experience, do not be discouraged. Try again a week later.

Keep up your aqua yoga practice as your baby grows, whenever you go swimming in the months and years to come. It is one of the simplest and best forms of exercise, contributing to the prevention of sickness and a feeling of total wellbeing as well as the promotion of good health for your family as a whole.

80 Water stretches with your baby

Postnatal stretches in water can be practised with your baby. You can hold your baby safely with both hands under the arms at first and then with one arm only. It is relatively easy to hold your baby against your body, facing out, with one of your arms across her chest extending to hold her arm between your thumb and index finger. Make sure you hold your baby in the most relaxed way you can and, whenever possible, allow her to find her own buoyancy in the water as well as relying on the support you give her.

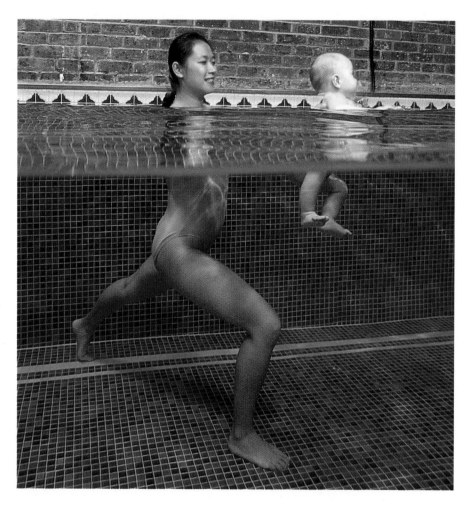

◁ **1** Many classic yoga poses can be done in water with your baby as part of your postnatal routine. Having your legs in the water gives you a stable and supple base from which to stretch and tone your body in the posture. Practising the warrior pose with your baby gives you strength and stamina that are communicated to her too. Extend your back leg and breathe as deeply as you can in your abdominal muscles on a strong base.

81 Relaxed floating with baby on board

Floating with your baby on your body is a marvellous feeling that completes all your practice of aqua yoga during pregnancy. When you are able to stretch back in the water and relax, if your baby is happy, let her lie freely on you, ready to hold her if needed only. You can also splash water gently on her body, which most babies find pleasurable. The more relaxed you are as you float, the better the experience for both of you.

You may ask your partner or a friend to give you support as you lower yourself in the water holding your baby, in the same way that you learnt to get into the position for Floating Relaxation. If you are on your own in a pool with a bar, you can use your feet under the bar as a departure point while you settle your baby on your body before taking your feet off to float. You can also have your baby resting on a float on top of you as you float on your back in the water, holding on to the sides of the board or to your baby's body on the board. In this case, your baby can be on her back, as described previously, or on her front, facing you. This may give you more confidence and some babies like it too. The body of a baby on a float will, however, be less immersed in the water than when resting on your body as you float, and you must make sure that the ambient temperature is high enough for comfort.

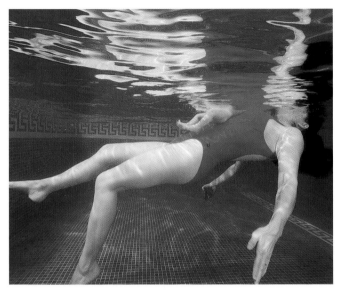

△ Most young babies enjoy lying on their backs on their mothers' bodies and you may experience sensations of rest similar to those felt during your pregnancy relaxation in water, except that now your baby is outside rather than inside. The freer you are in water, the more enjoyable the relaxation is for you both.

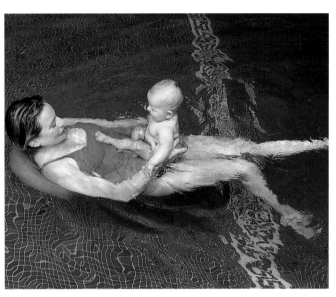

△ At first, even if you can float, the idea of your baby falling off may cause you to tense up. It may therefore be best to start with a long woggle or even two woggles under your arms, which allow you to have your two hands free to support your baby gently on the sides of her body.

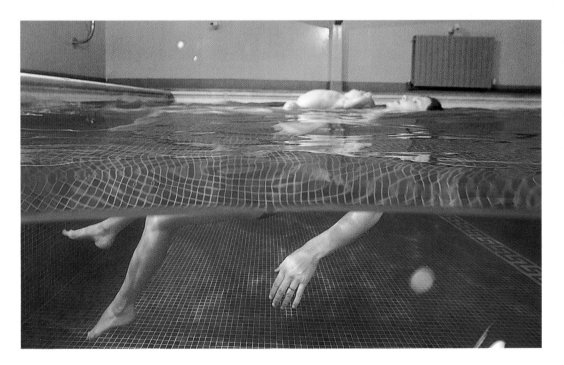

◁ At first you may prefer one foot to remain close to the pool floor to give you a feeling of security. However, if you can relax without any support with your baby on your body, then do so, as your baby is sensitive to the movement of your body and will be happy to enjoy the freedom water gives, yet be in close contact with you.

Water relief before and after birth

Aqua yoga exercises can be used to relieve backache in pregnancy. They also prove invaluable in soothing and treating the pelvic floor or your abdominal muscles after a Caesarean section.

At some point during your pregnancy you are likely to experience a form of backache. It is due mainly to the relaxation of your ligaments and joints in the pelvis that stretch you open, or to the destabilization of your sacroiliac joints (where your pelvis meets the lower spine) due to the increased weight of your growing baby when you walk or stand. Sometimes the pressure of your enlarged uterus may affect your sciatic nerves and cause acute pain. If your discomfort is constant and impairing, consult a doctor. Most common backache in pregnancy, however, responds well to yoga and even better to aqua yoga. In the buoyant environment of water, you can soothe your sore back and tone the muscles that will enable you to keep your spine aligned as you grow to full term. Regular aqua yoga will prevent any re-occurence.

The most soothing exercises are those in which you kneel or bend your knees and, if you are a swimmer, the leg movement of backstroke. All the hip rolls and loops will help you keep backache at bay once the pain has receded. After birth, aqua breathing will help you to heal and tone your perineum and pelvic floor, as well as the muscles of the lower abdomen. If you have had a Caesarean section, some postnatal aqua yoga twists and stretches will be most beneficial, while deep breathing can help to heal the scar tissue.

82 Backache in pregnancy

A great deal of backache in pregnancy is due to posture. Aligning your body in stretches with your knees bent and your back straight often helps to improve your posture and allows you to breathe more deeply, oxygenating the back muscles. Do the postures slowly, lowering your body in the water as much as you can and extending both your inhalations and your exhalations with each practice. If aqua yoga relieves your backache in two or three sessions at the pool, do not stop practising the postures that have helped you, as they continue to be effective in a preventive way. When you go to the pool with backache, be careful with draughts when you get out of the pool and make sure you have a large towel to wrap yourself in. If you have lower backache at any stage of pregnancy, here is a suggested sequence.

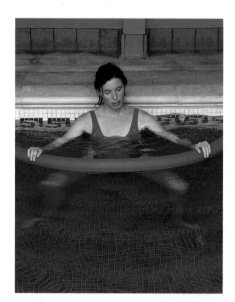

△ **1** From hip circle to full stretch: stand holding on to a bar or a woggle and practice Hip Circles (18). Try all the different circular movements you can make with your pelvis until you find one that particularly stretches and soothes your back. Then practise this one focusing on your breathing for a few minutes. You may find that the next time you go to the pool, you may need a slightly different hip circle.

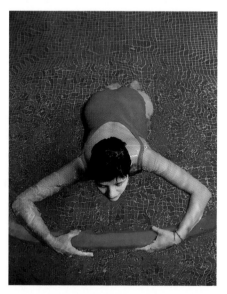

△ **2** To do a kneeling bend-stretch, place a woggle under your arms and lean forwards as you lower your bent knees in the water. If the pool is shallow enough, kneel on the pool floor.

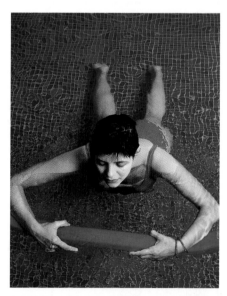

△ **3** Inhale, and as you exhale, allow your relaxed legs to extend back on the bottom of the pool, letting yourself drop as you hold on to the woggle. Then bend your knees again to return to your starting position and repeat this movement with the flow of the breath a few times, aiming at being more relaxed in it each time. The gentle contrast between the bending and stretching of your legs is particularly helpful with sciatic pain.

83 Healing the pelvic floor

Water is healing after giving birth and you have probably used baths at home to soothe your perineum if you had a tear or an episiotomy. It has been found, through controlled experiments, that a drop of lavender essential oil in the bath makes it even more effective. The first and main aqua yoga practice to rely on for better and speedier healing of the perineum is deep breathing sitting in water. Simply breathe at first and then lift your pelvic floor muscles using Reverse Breathing (54). This increases the blood circulation in the area and involves all the muscles together in their connection with the lower back and the lower abdominal muscles.

When you go to the pool there are two additional exercises that have proved to be helpful if you continue to be aware of your tear or cut, or if you have lost your vaginal tone or feel that your pelvic floor muscles remain weak.

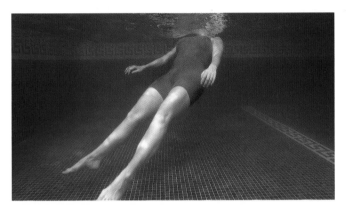

△ **1** Lie on your back in the water and stretch, trailing your extended legs. Use a woggle or board for support if you need to. Inhale and stretch more.

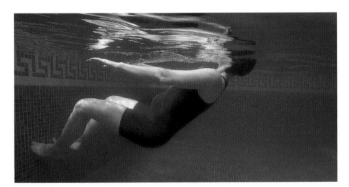

△ **2** As you exhale, bend your knees and bring them towards your body. Stretch again and let your legs drop, bend again, stretch again and so on. If your legs drop to the bottom of the pool, relax and stop, or start again from the beginning. If you get confident, you can combine this exercise with one of the aqua twists.

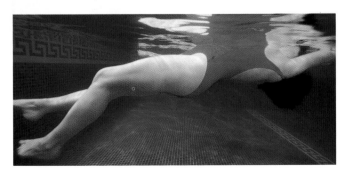

△ **3** Backstroke with wide leg movements, focusing on the stretching phase rather than on the opening of the knees, is also very effective.

84 After a Caesarean section

While all the postnatal aqua yoga stretches and adapted swimming are suitable if you practise them without exerting yourself after a Caesarean section, once you have healed your scar tissue with deep abdominal breathing and included Reverse Breathing (54), you can use aqua twists to breathe more deeply and tone your transverse abdominal muscles. Three of these twists can be practised together as a short sequence. Include them particularly in your postnatal routine.

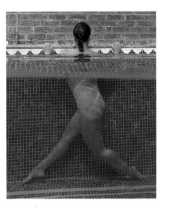

△ Wide twist, standing against the pool wall (64).

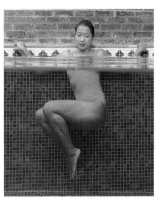

△ Twist-roll-bend (65).

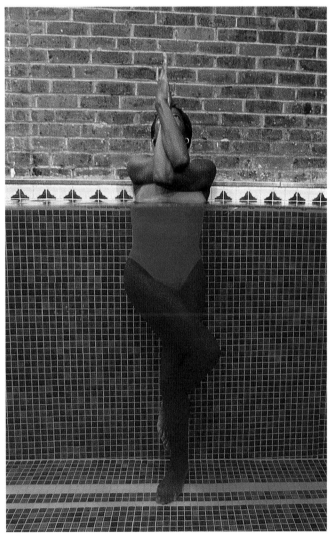

△ Eagle pose, legs only at first, then with the arms (66).

Useful addresses

United Kingdom

Promotion and supply of waterbirth pools

Active Birth Centre
25 Bickerton Road
London N19 5JT
Tel: 020 7561 9006

Splashdown Waterbirth Services
17 Wellington Terrace
Harrow on the Hill
Middlesex HA1 3EP
Tel: 020 8422 9308

Swimming advice

Amateur Swimming Association
Harold Fern House
Derby Square
Loughborough
Leicestershire LE11 0AL
Tel: 01509 618700

*The Alexander Technique applied
to swimming*

Aqua Development Programme
the Laboratory Health Club and Spa
The Avenue
Muswell Hill
London N10 2QJ
Tel: 020 8482 3000
www.art of swimming.com

*For details of aqua yoga classes (antenatal and
postnatal) and a supply of water woggles*

Birthlight
7 Essex Close
Cambridge CB4 2DW
Tel: 01223 362288
www.birthlight.com

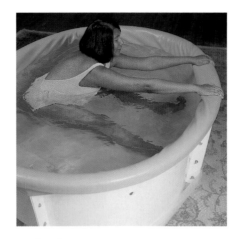

United States

**Global Maternal/Child Health
Association Ltd**
PO Box 1400
Wilsonville OR 97070
Tel. 503 682 3600
Fax. 503 682 3434
www.waterbirth.org
email: waterbirth@aol.com

Monadnock OB GYN Associates
454 Old Street Road
Peterborough
NH 03458
www.waterbirth.com

Citizens for Midwifery
PO Box 82227
Athens
GA 30608-2227
www.cfmidwifery.org

Supply of water woggles

**Rothama International Corp.
(Sprint Athletics)**
St. Louis Obispo
PO Box 3840
CA 93403
Tel: 800 235 2156

Useful books

The Teaching of Swimming, Amateur Swimming Association.

The Waterbirth Book, Balaskas, Janet and Y. Gordon (Thorsons, 1992)

Yoga for Pregnancy, Barbira Freedman, Françoise and D. Hall (Ward Lock, 1998)

Postnatal Yoga, Barbira Freedman, Françoise and D. Hall (Lorenz Books, 2000)

Waterbirth: an attitude to care, Garland, Dianne (Books for Midwives Press, second edition, 2000)

Total Immersion: the revolutionary way to swim better, faster and easier, Laughlin, Terry. (Simon & Schuster 1996)

The Waterbirth Handbook: the gentle art of waterbirthing, Lichy, Roger and E. Herzberg. (Gateway Books, 1993)

Water and Sexuality, Odent, Michel. (Arkana, 1990)

Swimming for Life: the therapy of swimming, Russsell, Ronald. (Pelham Books/Stephen Green, 1989)

The Art of Swimming, Shaw, Stephen and A. D'Angour. (Ashgrove Publishing, 1998)

Yoga and Health, Yesudian, S. and E. Haich. (Unwin Paperbacks, 1986)

From the author

My most special gratitude goes to my father: he took me swimming as a small child in the Loire near our home in France and his advanced yoga practice was an inspiration. Swimming coaches and yoga teachers from all over the world, too many to be named but all to be thanked, imparted the knowledge that I have drawn on in developing aqua yoga. Thanks to my own four, now grown, "water babies" who patiently shared long practice sessions.

Access to warm pools in Cambridge has been invaluable for *Birthlight* aqua yoga classes since the 1980's. My warmest thanks go to Geoff Barnes for his impeccable upkeep of the Windmill School pool and his great heart and also to Ruscha, whose beautiful pool at The Wood provided an ideal, conducive atmosphere to convey the power of water in pregnancy. Joanne and Nick also kindly let us use their pool in London. Thanks to Christine Hanscomb and her team: Zena, Russell and Jonas, who spared no effort to produce beautiful photographs. Sue Duckworth contributed more than her stylist's skills. The gentle yet firm coordination that Debra Mayhew conjured up as the editor at all stages in the making of this book was truly the X factor.

Aqua yoga has grown with the help of many friends and advisers of *Birthlight*. Thanks in particular to Sally Lomas, Tricia Beaumont and Louise Pivcevic for their assistance in teaching and, last but not least, to all the pregnant women and new mothers whose feedback has been essential to continue deepening my understanding of yoga in water.

The models

With many thanks to the models for their enthusiasm and patience:

Myriam Baldor with George and Matthew; Kristin Cauvas; Patricia Cave; Pam Ha-Stevenson with Joshua; Alison Gilderdale with Alice and Luke; Susanna Glimmezveen; Sarah Gostick with Isobel; Rowena Guzy; Stacia Keogh; Yane Lassen; Lisa Messenger with Kate; Meena Singh with Shanti Lara; Hester Tingey with Bathsheba; Sabine Ulmer-Lake; Safuriat Yesufu with Morton.

Index

Alternate nostril breathing 16,17,55
amniotic fluid 9
antenatal aqua yoga 18–41
    about the exercises 16–17
    aims 16
    aqua breathing 20–21
    aqua yoga poses 34–5
    aqua yoga together 40–41
    arms and shoulders 32–3
    dynamic stretches 36–7
    energetic stretches 38–9
    hip openers 26–7
    hip rolls and loops 24–5
    knee and hip circles 30–31
    kneel open and swing 28–9
    pelvic floor muscles 23
    spinal alignment and awareness 22
antenatal swimming 42–9
    adapted backstroke 46–7
    adapted breaststroke swimming 44–5
    freestyle swimming 48–9
anxiety 54
aqua breathing
    Aqua breathing for non-swimmers 20
    Submerged breathing 21
    Supported breathing stretches 21
Aqua yoga breaststroke 45
archer pose 24,29,65
    Kneeling archer pose 29
arms and shoulders
    Arm twists 32–3
    Standing and supported breaststroke 33
    Water sun wheels 32
asanas 34
asthma 10,14
Ayurveda 56
baby
    and bathtime 17
    foetal heart rate 12,61
    newborn baby 69
    and waterbirth 60–61
back
    Back bend stretch 37
    Full back stretch 36–7

muscles 17
    problems 10,12,24,30,69
back crawl 46
    Front and back crawl 48
Back rowing 46
backstroke 48
    asymmetrical backstroke 46
    Back rowing 46
    Backstroke leg circles 47
    "English backstroke" 46
    symmetrical backstroke 46
bathtime 17
bearing down 68
birthing pool 60,61,62,64,65,66
blood, oxygenated 13,64
blood pressure 12,53
brainwaves 54
breaststroke 44
    Aqua yoga breaststroke 45
    Standing and supported breaststroke 33
    Water-boatwoman 44
breathing 10,11,16,17,28,44
    Alternate nostril breathing 16,17,55
    Aqua breathing for non-swimmers 20
    aqua breathing for waterbirthing 66–7
    the breath of life 52–3
    Breathe yourself open 63
    Breathing dives with relaxation 52–3
    Breathing through your contractions in water 67
    and pain relief 51
    Reverse breathing 72
    Submerged breathing 21
    Supported breathing stretches 21
    toning with 72
butterfly stroke 48,49

Caesarean section 10,63,72,93
cardio-vascular function 10,13
cervix 64,65,67
chest muscles 32
chlorine 14,15
circulatory system 10
contractions 64,65,68,69
    Breathing through your contractions in water 67
    relaxation between 66
crawl 48
    see also back crawl; front crawl
Cross-arms 73

dehydration 15,66
delta brainwaves 54
diaphragm, effective use of 44
dives
    Breathing dives with relaxation 52–3
    Dolphin dives 49,88
dopplers, submersible 61
drifting 56
Drops 22,55
endorphins 54,66
"English backstroke" 46
equipment for practice 15

Float-drop 63
Floating butterfly pose 35
floating relaxation 9,17,20,21
    the benefits of relaxation 54

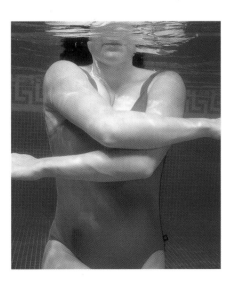

drifting 56
Floating relaxation before birth 63
Relaxation with a partner 55
relaxation and release 56
supported relaxation 54
theta brainwaves 54
using supports 56
With One Woggle Under the Knees, Holding On 56
With One Woggle Under the Knees, Letting Go 57
With Two Woggles, Holding On 57
Floating tree pose 35
floats 15,56
foam boards 34
Free standing in the water 22
freestyle swimming
Dolphin dives 49
Front and back crawl 48
Full back stretch 36-7
"fun noodles" (see woggles)

goggles 15

harmony 9,11
Healing the pelvic floor 93
heart, and labour 32,64
Hip circles 30-31
Hip loop forward and back 25
hip openers
Open stretch and pelvic swing 27
Opening steps 26
Russian squats 26-7
Hip rolls and figures-of-eight 24
Hip wheel 25
hydrotherapy pools 14

immune system 10

Joints
flexibility 26
Joint floating stretch 41
problems 10

Knee circles 30
Knee-bent variations 65
kneeling
Kneel down and turn 28
Kneeling archer pose 20
Kneeling close and lift 73
Kneeling or half kneeling (for waterbirth) 69
Swing from kneeling to squatting & back again 29

labour 10
and the heart 32
pain relief 13,51,59,61,66
preparation for 26
"second stage" 68
see also waterbirth
labour partner 55
Leg circles on the back 40
ligaments 10
pelvic 11,22
lymph nodes 46

massage in water 10
miscarriages 56
muscles 11

abdominal 12,17,28
chest 32
isokinetic contraction of 13
mobility 10
pelvic floor 17,23,66,72
strength 10
tone 10,13

"natural childbirth" 61
nose clips 20

Open stands, drops and hip swings 62
Open stretch and pelvic swing 27
Opening steps 26

pain relief in labour 13,51,59,61,66
pelvic exercise 13
Pelvic floor lift and release 23
pelvic floor muscles 17,23,66,72
Pelvic rolls and swings in the birthing pool 64
Pelvic swing, open stretch and 27
pelvis 11
perineum 23,65,68
placenta 69
postnatal aqua yoga 70-73
about the exercises 17
aims 17
closing the body 72-3
involving the baby 13
posture 11,12,13,24
practice
choosing a pool 14-15
equipment for practice 15
how to practise 15
pranayama 17
pratyahara 54
pregnancy 12-13
terminations 56
progesterone 26
prolactin 66
pulse rate 10
relaxation 9,13,16,17,20,26,34,35,41,46
between contractions 66
Breathing dives with relaxation 52-3
Relaxation with a partner 55

see also floating relaxation
Relaxed floating with baby on board 91
Relaxed roll stretch 39
Reverse breathing 72
Russian squats 26-7

safety 15,56
sciatica 30
sodium hypochloride 14
spinal aligment 17,22,74
Squat, semi-squat and supported standing 68
stamina 10,72
Standing and supported breaststroke 33
strength 10,72
Stretch-float (for waterbirth) 69
stretches
Back bend stretch 37
Bend stretch 81
Front and back stretch 80
Full back stretch 36-7
Knee-bent stretch 75
Leg stretch 75
Realigning the spine 74
Relaxed roll stretch 39
Water turtle 38-9
Submerged breathing 21
suppleness 10
Supported breathing stretches 21
swimming pools 14-15
Swing from kneeling to squatting and back again 29

temperature, water 14,15,64,66
toddlers 41
twists
Eagle pose 79
Extended twist 82
Narrow twists 76
Snake bend 83
Twist-roll-bend 78
Wide twist 77

uterus
and contractions 66,67
supply of blood to 64

vagina
and the birth 68
tone 23
visualization 64

Warrior balance 34
water
and giving birth 68
an ideal medium for yoga 9,19,34
temperature 14,15,64,66
Water stretches with your baby 90
Water sun wheels 32
Water turtle 38-9
Water-boatwoman 44
waterbirth 13,58-69
aqua breathing for waterbirthing 66-7
aqua yoga for labour 64-5
the benefits of water in labour and birth 60-63,68
Stretch-float 69
woggles 15,34

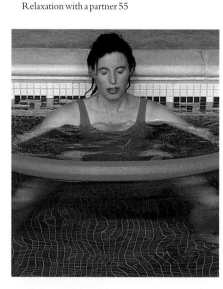